Designing Your Longevity

A Personalized Blueprint for Thriving Longer with Energy, Purpose, and Vitality

Maria L. Ellis, BBA, MBA

Washington, DC, USA

Published 2025

DISCLAIMER

DEDICATION

To the bold believers, the ones who know deep in their hearts that life's most extraordinary chapters are not behind them, but still ahead. To the dreamers and doers of every age who choose growth over comfort, hope over fear, and purpose over resignation.

This book, *Designing Your Longevity: A Personalized Blueprint for Thriving Longer with Energy, Purpose, and Vitality*, is a love letter to possibility—and it is especially dedicated to my beloved family and cherished friends. Your unwavering support, contagious laughter, and timeless wisdom breathe life into my every endeavor. You remind me daily that we are meant to thrive, not just survive.

And to future generations: may you rise in a world that celebrates limitless vitality, embraces purpose as a way of life, and dares to believe that aging is not an ending—but a magnificent beginning.

— Maria L. Ellis, BBA, MBA

TABLE OF CONTENTS

FOREWORD

By Dr. Graham F. Whitfield, MD, PhD, FICS

Clinical Associate Professor of Orthopedic Surgery
(Nova Southeastern University)
Current Position - Palm Beach Orthopedic Specialists

As a physician and surgeon with over four decades of experience in orthopedic medicine, I've had the privilege of treating thousands of patients from all walks of life. And if there is one constant across those years, it is this: our healthspan—the quality of the years we live—is just as important, if not more so, than our lifespan.

The prevailing assumption in modern medicine has long been that aging is a gradual, irreversible decline—a march toward fragility and dysfunction. But we now understand that this trajectory is not a biological inevitability. It is often the result of lifestyle choices, environmental stressors, and, most crucially, a lack of early, intentional intervention. *Designing Your Longevity: A Personalized Blueprint for Thriving Longer with Energy, Purpose, and Vitality* provides both the evidence and the inspiration to rethink that path.

This book offers a compelling synthesis of the science behind healthy aging, including developments in cellular biology, inflammation control, biomechanics, and neurocognitive resilience. It challenges the reader to shift from a reactive approach to aging—waiting until something breaks—to a proactive strategy rooted in prevention, movement, mindset, and personalized care.

What sets this book apart is its practicality. The author has translated complex science into accessible, actionable insights. Whether you're a busy professional, an active retiree, or someone simply curious about optimizing your later years, this guide provides a clear and motivating roadmap.

As a medical doctor with a PhD in organic chemistry, I am particularly impressed by the rigorous attention paid to both emerging scientific research and the timeless principles of holistic well-being. But perhaps even more important is the human element woven throughout this work: the call to live not just longer, but with purpose, connection, and vitality.

If you are ready to invest in your health not just for the next year—but for the next decade and beyond—this book is a timely and invaluable companion.

—

Graham F. Whitfield, MD, PhD, FICS
Clinical Assistant Professor, Orthopedic Surgery
Palm Beach Orthopedic Specialist

CHAPTER 1:
THE WEIGHT OF TIME
AND LONELINESS

*"Aging is not the end of the road; it is simply a turn
leading to a new path waiting to be explored."*
— Maria L. Ellis, BBA, MBA

At seventy-two, Sofia found herself standing at a precipice she had never foreseen. She had spent decades as a devoted schoolteacher, shaping young minds with patience and care. She had raised four children, pouring love and wisdom into them, nurturing their dreams while sacrificing her own. Her home had once been a sanctuary of warmth, laughter, and purpose. She remembered one particular spring morning, years ago, when her youngest daughter, Elena, had stood on a stool in their sunlit kitchen, helping her knead dough for sweet bread. Flour dusted the countertops like soft snow, and laughter echoed through the room as music played from the old radio in the corner. "Mama," Elena had said, her small hands pressing into the dough, "when I grow up, I want to be just like you." Sofia had smiled, brushing a strand of hair from her daughter's cheek, her heart swelling with quiet joy. That moment – simple, fleeting – had felt like forever. But now, that purpose had dissolved into the stillness that surrounded her.

Her children had long since grown, their lives now orbiting careers, spouses, and children of their own. Though they called when they could and visited on holidays, it was never enough to fill the vast emptiness she felt. The once-familiar sounds of life – the giggles of grandchildren, the hum of conversation over dinner, the comforting chaos of a full house – had been replaced by an eerie silence that stretched endlessly through the halls of her apartment.

Each morning, she struggled not just to rise from bed but to find a reason to do so. Her arthritis gnawed at her joints, making simple movements an exhausting ordeal. Walking to the grocery store, something she had once done effortlessly, now felt like an insurmountable challenge. The city she had navigated with such confidence in her younger years now seemed unwelcoming, its hurried pace leaving her behind.

Yet, the physical pain was nothing compared to the weight of time itself. When she looked in the mirror, she barely recognized the woman staring back at her. Her once-bright eyes now held the heaviness of years gone by. Her skin, once smooth and radiant, bore the inevitable traces of age. She saw in herself not just the passage of time but the fading of a life she had worked so hard to build. Maybe you've felt it too – the subtle shift when people stop really seeing you. The way conversations glide past you at family gatherings, or how clerks and waiters seem to look right through you. There's the quiet stiffness in your joints, the slower rise from a chair, and the moment of pause before facing your reflection, wondering when your eyes began to look so tired. And beneath it all, a question you rarely say out loud: *Is this it?* Like Sofia, you may be carrying the ache of time and the quiet grief of a life poured into others – noble, necessary, even beautiful – but never fully your own.

She had always believed that retirement would bring peace – a time to savor the life she had spent decades constructing. Instead, she felt invisible. Discarded. The world that had once needed her had moved on, seemingly without a backward glance. She had given everything – to her family, her students, her community – and now she questioned: Had she given too much? Had she lost herself in the process?

Loneliness became her constant companion. She spent hours by the window, watching the world rush past, feeling like a spectator in a life she no longer belonged to. The friendships that had once sustained her had either faded with time or succumbed to the inevitable distance of busy lives. She longed for connection, for a voice that broke the quiet, for a reminder that she still mattered.

More than anything, she feared not death, but the possibility of continuing to exist in this state – adrift, unseen, untethered. Was this truly all there was?

Something had to change. Deep inside, a flicker of defiance remained – a whisper that told her this couldn't be the end of her story. But where did she even begin? The weight of her past, the relentless ache in her body, and the silence of an empty home all seemed impossible to overcome.

Yet, as she sat in her chair by the window, watching the sun dip below the horizon, she allowed herself to wonder: *What if?*

What if there was still more waiting for her? What if you could redefine what it meant to age? What if this wasn't the closing chapter, but the start of something new?

Know that you are not alone. I have met so many women – strong, loving, giving – who one day wake up and wonder where their energy, their spark, and even their sense of self have gone. Like Sofia, they have given everything to everyone else and are now left wondering what's left for them. But I want you to know something important: this moment is not the end. It's a turning point. I have walked this road with others before, and I have seen the transformation that is possible when you begin to reclaim your health, your purpose, and your joy. Don't worry

– I have got you! We are going to take this journey togeth-er, one hopeful step at a time.

CHAPTER 2:
THE EVOLUTION OF
LONGEVITY – MY JOURNEY
AND THE PATH FORWARD

*"Longevity is not about adding years to your life;
it's about adding life to your years."*
— Maria L. Ellis, BBA, MBA

It was a quiet Sunday morning, the kind I used to cherish – coffee in hand, watching the sunrise from the balcony at my oceanfront apartment, sunlight pouring through the windows, a sense of peace. But that morning, something was different. I had just gotten off the phone with a dear friend, Ursula, who lives in my apartment building, someone I hadn't spoken to in weeks.

She had always prided herself on staying active. For years, she taught a gentle yoga class at the community center, guiding others through breath and movement with calm assurance. But now, even walking up a flight of stairs left her breathless. "I stopped teaching," she confessed to me, her voice barely above a whisper. "I just don't have the energy anymore." Her doctor had recently diagnosed her with early-stage heart disease – plaque quietly building up in her arteries like time layering itself in her body. "I guess this is just part of getting old," she said, almost apologetically, as if aging were something to be ashamed of.

That moment stayed with me – not just because of Ursula's diagnosis, but because of her resignation. Too many women like her – like us – begin to believe that fading is inevitable. That the best is behind us. But what if that isn't true? What if science, technology, and a new understanding of the human body are rewriting the rules of aging? And what if you could step into that next chapter – not with fear, but with purpose?

I hung up and sat in silence for a long time. That conversation echoed in my head. I couldn't shake the weight of it – not just her words but the resignation behind them. I realized then that something inside me had shifted too.

I had written my first book on longevity to spark hope, to offer science-based tools and stories that could inspire reinvention at any age. But that morning, I understood that one book wasn't enough. The science had evolved. The stories had deepened. And so had I. I had grown – emotionally, physically, and spiritually – reshaping my own understanding of what it means to age with vitality and purpose. Longevity isn't just about adding years to life – it's about adding life to years, especially when it feels like the world is quietly asking you to shrink, to slow down, to disappear. I decided to reject that quiet fading and instead crown myself the Queen of Energy, Vitality, and Love.

I looked at my own routines – the way I move, eat, think, rest, connect – and realized I had quietly built a new blueprint. A sustainable way to thrive, not just survive. And more than ever, I wanted to share that with others.

That morning became the moment I knew I had to write this sequel. Not as a follow-up, but as a continuation of a movement. This book isn't about chasing youth – it's about choosing energy and vitality. And you don't need to do it alone. I have lived this. I am living it now. And I will walk beside you every step of the way.

That morning lit a fire in me – not just to write, but to live even more intentionally. I began looking at my own daily habits through a new lens. What was really working? What made me feel energized, clear-minded, and strong? And what needed to evolve?

I started with movement. Not intense workouts or punishing routines, but consistent, life-giving motion. I committed to walking every morning – just thirty minutes in the fresh air, often with a podcast or calming playlist. I added strength training twice a week, not to sculpt a perfect body, but to support the one I have – to keep my bones strong, my posture upright, and my independence intact. I wanted to be able to carry my own groceries, climb the stairs without holding the railing, reach for a dish on the top shelf, or get up from the floor after playing with my grandchild – on my own terms, without hesitation or fear. I danced in my kitchen, in my living room, whenever the spirit moved me. Because movement should be joyful. That joy alone is healing.

Next, I revisited how I nourished myself. I stopped seeing food as a set of restrictions and started embracing it as a source of healing and energy. I used to crave milk chocolate – the sweeter, the better – but over time, I found myself drawn to the rich complexity of bitter dark chocolate. It surprised me how my taste shifted as my mindset and body began to change. I started asking a powerful question: How can I love myself through what I eat? I focused on whole, colorful foods – lots of greens, berries, healthy fats, and clean proteins. I gave my body what it needed to repair and thrive, not just to get through the day. I also became more mindful of when I ate. Intermittent fasting became a gentle practice – twelve to fourteen hours between dinner and breakfast – giving my body time to rest and reset.

Sleep, I realized, is not a luxury – it's a longevity tool. I stopped glorifying busyness and started protecting my rest. I turned off screens earlier, embraced rituals like herbal tea and soft music, and created a bedroom space that felt like a sanctuary. My sleep improved, and so did everything else

– my focus, mood, and even my skin.

Longevity isn't just physical. I cultivated mental and emotional resilience through daily meditation, journaling, and gratitude practice. Even five minutes a day of stillness helped me tune into my body and mind. I found myself calmer, more centered, and less reactive. I also reached out more – to old friends, to community groups, to new opportunities. I began attending biohacking conferences, exploring cutting-edge wellness centers, and surrounding myself with people who were just as curious and committed to living fully as I was. Connection is one of the most overlooked ingredients of longevity. We need one another to stay well. These experiences expanded not only my knowledge but also my belief in what's possible at any age.

This chapter isn't about perfection – it's about momentum. I didn't change everything overnight. I just chose to take the next right step every day. And those steps added up. So now, as you turn this page, I want you to remember: this is possible for you, too. Whether you have already started your journey or feel like you're just waking up to it – you're not too late, and it's not too hard. You don't have to become someone new. You just need to reconnect with the person you were always meant to be.

Let's begin by redefining aging. Aging is a paradox. It is both a privilege and a challenge, a journey marked by wisdom and yet, at times, accompanied by a sense of loss. At seventy-five, I find myself reflecting deeply on what it means to age well. I have lived a full and vibrant life – I have built businesses, nurtured relationships, traveled the world, and pursued my passions. Yet, I also feel the weight of time. My body is not as forgiving as it once was, and when I look in the mirror, I no longer see the youthful face I once knew. I won't deny it – sometimes that realization makes me sad.

But here is what I've learned: longevity is not about looking young – it's about feeling strong, energetic, and capable of living life to the fullest. It's about redefining what it means to age, moving past society's obsession with youth, and instead, embracing a science-backed approach to optimizing our health, extending our lifespan, and – most importantly – improving our quality of life.

This chapter is deeply personal. It is the story of my own transformation, my struggles with health challenges, and the cutting-edge strategies I have adopted to rewrite my future. It is also a roadmap for you, the reader – because longevity is not reserved for a select few. It is a choice, a commitment, and a way of life. Let's embark on this journey together.

Reframing Beauty and Embracing Vitality

One of the greatest shifts I had to make in my longevity journey was moving beyond society's definition of beauty. For years, I equated youth with attractiveness, and aging with decline. But I've come to realize that true beauty is not about wrinkle-free skin or a flawless figure – it is about confidence, wisdom, and vitality.

I have seen women in their eighties and nineties radiate a presence that commands attention – not because they look young, but because they exude an energy that draws people in. That is the kind of beauty I now strive for.

How I Reclaimed My Radiance at Seventy-Five

I changed my definition of beauty. Instead of chasing youth, I began focusing on how I felt. Was I strong? Was I vibrant? Was I living with purpose? The more I focused on my inner health, the more it reflected outwardly. I embraced the idea that beauty is how you carry yourself – your posture, the way you dress, your enthusiasm for life.

I started a transformative self-care routine. I introduced biohacking tools into my daily regimen to support cellular health and rejuvenation. Red Light Therapy became a game-changer for me – it stimulates collagen production, improves skin tone, and even enhances energy at a mito-chondrial level. I also began taking targeted supplements like EPA and DHA capsules to support overall cellular health and promote my body's natural collagen production. Eicosapentaenoic acid (EPA) and docosahexaenoic acid (DHA) are omega-3 fatty acids primarily found in fatty fish like salmon, mackerel, and sardines. They play a vital role in reducing inflammation, supporting heart and brain health, and promoting healthy skin and joints. Studies also suggest they help stimulate collagen production, which can enhance skin elasticity and slow visible signs of aging. Facial massage and red light therapy became part of my biweekly routine, not just for appearance, but as rituals of care and vitality. Over the years, facial exercises and lymphatic massage have improved my circulation and given my face a natural, lifted look.

I embraced my presence. Instead of hiding behind neutral colors, I began wearing vibrant tones that made me feel alive. I focused on maintaining good posture – standing tall not only made me look more confident, but it also improved my energy levels. I made a conscious effort to engage with people, make eye contact, and share my wisdom. There is nothing more magnetic than a person who carries themselves with purpose.

One of the most exciting developments in longevity science is Red Light Therapy (RLT). This technology uses specific wavelengths of red and near-infrared light to penetrate deep into the skin, stimulating mitochondrial activity and promoting collagen production. The result? Improved skin texture, reduced inflammation, and increased energy.

Biohacking My Health and Reversing Age-Related Decline

The body is a complex system, and aging is not just about appearance – it's about cellular function, metabolic efficiency, and overall resilience. As I delved deeper into longevity science, I realized that the key to aging well is preventing cellular damage and optimizing repair mechanisms.

I targeted nutrition: Eating for Longevity. I transitioned to a nutrient-dense diet focused on whole, anti-inflammatory foods. I began incorporating intermittent fasting, allowing my body time to repair itself through a process called autophagy, which removes damaged cells and promotes regeneration. I prioritized protein intake to preserve muscle mass – one of the most important factors for longevity.

Supplements and Advanced Therapies

- NMN (Nicotinamide Mononucleotide) – This supplement supports NAD+ levels, essential for cellular energy and DNA repair.
- Resveratrol – A powerful antioxidant found in red wine that has been linked to longevity and cardiovascular health.
- Mitochondrial Support – I started taking CoQ10 and PQQ, which enhance cellular energy production.

As we age, hormone levels decline, leading to fatigue, loss of muscle mass, and cognitive issues. I worked with a specialist to optimize my hormone levels through bioidentical hormone therapy. Addressing thyroid function was a game-changer for my metabolism and energy levels. One of the most fascinating longevity interventions I have explored is Hyperbaric Oxygen Therapy. This treatment increases oxygen levels in the bloodstream, promoting neurogenesis (new brain cell growth) and enhancing cognitive function.

Strength and Movement – The Key to Staying Independent

As I aged, I noticed that maintaining muscle mass and bone density was critical for longevity. Frailty is one of the biggest risk factors for aging-related decline, leading to falls, fractures, and loss of independence.

Detoxing the Body, Mind, and Spirit: Clearing the Path for Vitality

Before we can regenerate, we must release. One of the most essential – but often overlooked – steps in the longevity journey is detoxification. Over the years, our bodies accumulate waste, toxins, and stressors from processed foods, environmental pollution, pharmaceutical residue, and even our own negative thought patterns. These burdens compromise our energy, cloud our minds, and impair our body's natural ability to heal.

Stop Poisoning the Body

Longevity isn't just about what we add to our lives – it's about what we remove. Clean eating and supplementation are powerful, but we must also examine what we continue to consume, both physically and emotionally. Every choice matters: the foods we eat, the air we breathe, the products we use, the habits we reinforce.

When I committed to stop poisoning my body – with chemicals, processed food, excessive caffeine, and even certain toxic relationships – I began to experience clarity and vitality on a new level. Detoxification is not punishment – it's liberation.

Cleanse to Reclaim Your Energy

Through targeted cleansing practices – hydration, fasting, herbal teas, saunas, breathwork, and lymphatic movement – I began to feel lighter, clearer, and more alive. Detox isn't a trend; it's a return to our natural state of balance. The body knows how to heal if we simply create the conditions for it.

Release Toxic Thoughts and Habits

Cleansing isn't just physical. Our thoughts, emotions, and subconscious programming can be just as toxic as chemicals in our food. I began to notice how old patterns

– self-doubt, guilt, anxiety – kept me locked in a low vibrational state. Letting go of these internal poisons was as critical as detoxifying my body.

Create Empowering Habits and a New Identity

Lasting change comes from identity. I didn't just want to feel better – I wanted to be someone new. I began developing habits that supported the woman I wanted to become: consistent movement, uplifting conversations, nutrient-rich meals, mindfulness practices, and moments of joy. Over time, these became automatic. They weren't chores – they were expressions of who I had become.

And so I claimed a new identity: I am the Queen of Energy, Vitality, and Love. What title would you give yourself today?

This is not just a mantra – it's my truth. It guides the way I live, the choices I make, the energy I share. And you can do the same. You can release the old and step into the new. You can become the King or Queen of your own vibrant, purpose-driven life.

How I Stay Strong and Mobile at Seventy-Five

Strength training and resistance exercises. Lifting weights three to four times a week has reversed muscle loss, improved my balance, and increased my metabolism. I focus on compound movements like squats, deadlifts, and push-ups. I practice yoga and stretching to keep my joints mobile and prevent stiffness. Walking remains my favorite form of exercise – daily movement is the simplest yet most powerful longevity tool. I must confess that I have not yet started incorporating cold plunges and infrared sauna therapy, which have been shown to reduce inflammation, improve circulation, and enhance recovery.

Aging Is a Choice – A New Path Forward

Longevity is no longer a mystery – it is a science. And what I have discovered is that aging well is a choice. Every day, we have the opportunity to nourish our bodies, challenge our minds, and embrace the latest advancements in health and technology to extend not just our lifespan, but our health span – the years we live in vibrant, thriving health.

I have rewritten the narrative of my own aging, and so can you.

The path forward is clear: Reframe your mindset – aging is an opportunity, not a decline. Adopt longevity-focused nutrition and biohacking strategies. Prioritize movement and strength. Embrace cutting-edge therapies that optimize cellular function. The best years are not behind us. They are right here, waiting for us to claim them. Are you ready to redefine aging?

Let's start by thinking about these reflection questions:

- What was your "wake-up call?"
- Was there a moment recently – big or small – when you felt something needed to change in how you live, move, or take care of yourself?
- How do you feel in your body right now?
- Are there aches, fatigue, or moments of low energy that you've been ignoring or accepting as "normal?"
- What one daily habit could bring you more vitality?
- Think small – could it be a morning walk, a healthier breakfast, a five-minute stretch, or turning off screens earlier?
- What brings you joy that you haven't done in a while?
- Dancing? Gardening? Laughing with a friend? How can you invite more of that into your life starting this week?
- Who can you reach out to for connection or support?
- Is there someone you have been meaning to call or a group you have been curious about joining?

Connection is healing – what step can you take?

As I reflect on my own journey, I realize that true longevity is not measured by the ticking of the clock, but by the richness of each moment lived with purpose, vitality, and love. My transformation has been fueled by a willingness to embrace change, to explore cutting-edge strategies, and to continually reimagine what a full life can be. The path forward is clear: longevity is not merely about extending time, but about enhancing the quality of that time – through movement, mindfulness, connection, and science-driven innovation.

I invite you to walk this path with me, to become the architect of your future, and to remember that the greatest gift you can give yourself is not simply more years – but more life in every year.

CHAPTER 3:
NUTRITION FOR LONGEVITY – THE FOUNDATION OF A LONGER LIFE

"Let food be thy medicine and medicine be thy food."
— Hippocrates

Now that you've heard my story, let's look at how we'll redefine aging together. Over the next chapters, we'll dive into the core pillars of lasting vitality – starting with the choices you make every day. We'll explore how nutrition, movement, restorative sleep, stress management, and even cutting-edge breakthroughs in AI and science can extend not just your years, but the quality of those years. Think of each chapter as a building block in your longevity blueprint. And we begin with the most essential one: nutrition – the foundation of a longer, stronger life.

Nutrition is step one in our longevity journey because it underpins every other strategy we'll explore. When you fuel your body with the right foods, you create a solid foundation for everything else – better energy for movement, deeper sleep, improved mood, and greater resilience to stress. By getting your diet working for you, we make the next steps – like exercise, rest, and even advanced therapies – far more effective. This is where lasting transformation begins.

Reducing inflammation isn't just about avoiding chronic illness – it's about reclaiming your energy and your vitality. Less inflammation means steadier energy, clearer thinking, and more days where you feel truly alive. And more energy means more time spent being active with your loved ones, not just watching from the sidelines. Remember Sofia – sitting by the window, aching to be part of life again? These nutrition changes are how we shift that story. Imagine waking up clear-headed and strong, ready to take on your day with purpose. That's what this is really about – not just antioxidants or blood sugar levels, but ensuring you never feel invisible, tired, or stuck again. This is science in service of your freedom.

Food for Medicine

For centuries, civilizations have recognized the profound connection between food and health. Yet, in modern times, nutrition has been largely reduced to convenience – processed meals, quick fixes, and fast food have become the norm. While these choices provide temporary satisfaction, they come at a cost: chronic disease, inflammation, and accelerated aging.

The truth is what we eat determines how we age. Food is not just about sustenance; it is information that tells our cells how to function. Every bite we take influences our energy levels, metabolism, brain function, and even the rate at which our cells deteriorate.

I spent years eating whatever was easy, often choosing comfort foods over truly nourishing meals. I didn't realize that my declining energy, joint pain, and sluggishness were all linked to my diet. But once I made the connection, everything changed.

This chapter is about the power of food to transform our bodies, extend our health span, and even slow aging at a cellular level. By embracing a longevity-focused diet, we can not only add years to our lives but, more importantly, add life to our years.

Longevity is not just about genetics – it is about daily choices. Research shows that up to 80 percent of our lifespan is determined by lifestyle factors, with nutrition playing a central role.

People who live the longest, such as those in the Blue Zones – regions with the highest concentration of centenarians – share common dietary habits. Their diets are rich in whole, plant-based foods, healthy fats, and lean proteins, while being low in processed sugars and harmful additives. Watch out for common additives like artificial sweeteners (such as aspartame or sucralose) and food dyes (like Red 40 or Yellow 5), which can disrupt gut health and have been linked to inflammation and other health concerns. A quick tip: when reading ingredient labels, aim for products with short, recognizable ingredient lists – if you can't pronounce it or wouldn't cook with it at home, it's worth reconsidering.

The goal of longevity nutrition is simple: reduce inflammation, support cellular health, and nourish the body with the right nutrients. Here's how:

Antioxidants and Phytochemicals: The Body's Defense System

Oxidative stress is a major driver of aging. Over time, free radicals – unstable molecules – damage our cells and contribute to age-related diseases. Antioxidants neutralize these harmful molecules, reducing inflammation and slowing cellular damage. Key sources of antioxidants include polyphenols – found in berries, green tea, and dark chocolate, polyphenols protect against heart disease and support brain health. Carotenoids – present in carrots, sweet potatoes, and leafy greens, these compounds enhance eye health and reduce cancer risk – and flavonoids – found in citrus fruits, onions, and soy, flavonoids have anti-inflammatory properties that strengthen the immune system.

Some of my favorite superfoods include turmeric and

curcumin, which I love adding to my soups and stews for both their rich flavor and powerful anti-inflammatory benefits. A powerful anti-inflammatory that protects against neurodegenerative diseases like Alzheimer's. Spirulina and chlorella – rich in protein, vitamins, and minerals, these algae detoxify the body and support immune function.

Omega-3 fatty acids are essential for reducing inflammation, improving cognitive function, and protecting against heart disease. These healthy fats are found in fatty fish (salmon, mackerel, sardines), chia seeds, flaxseeds, and walnuts. Research shows that people with higher omega-3 levels live longer and have lower rates of neurodegenerative diseases.

The Mediterranean Diet: The Gold Standard for Longevity

The Mediterranean diet is one of the most well-researched dietary patterns linked to long life. It is based on fruits and vegetables – rich in fiber and antioxidants. Whole grains and legumes – support gut health and stable blood sugar. Healthy fats (olive oil, nuts, avocados) – reduce inflammation. Lean proteins (fish, poultry, plant-based sources) – maintain muscle mass and limited red meat and processed sugars – protect against disease.

Case Study: The Greek EPIC Study – Unlocking Longevity Through the Mediterranean Diet

For centuries, the people of the Mediterranean have enjoyed long, vibrant lives, fueled by a diet rich in fresh, whole foods and powerful, life-extending nutrients. But does science back up the benefits of this legendary way of eating? A landmark study – the Greek EPIC (European Prospective Investigation into Cancer and Nutrition) Study – tracked the health of over 22,000 adults in Greece, revealing astonishing findings: 25 percent lower mortality rate – participants who adhered closely to the Mediterranean diet were significantly less likely to die from all causes, proving that diet plays a crucial role in extending lifespan.

Fewer Cases of Heart Disease

Thanks to the diet's abundance of heart-protective omega-3s, healthy fats, and antioxidants, participants experienced reduced inflammation, lower cholesterol levels, and stronger cardiovascular health.

Lower Cancer Risk – rich in polyphenols, fiber, and anti-inflammatory compounds, the Mediterranean diet provided cellular protection against oxidative stress, reducing the likelihood of chronic diseases, including various cancers.

Sharper Minds and Lower Rates of Cognitive Decline

The diet's emphasis on brain-boosting foods like olive oil, fish, nuts, and leafy greens was linked to better cognitive function and a reduced risk of Alzheimer's and dementia. If you have ever worried about your memory slipping, this may give you hope.

The Greek EPIC Study reaffirmed what Mediterranean cultures have known for generations – food is not just fuel; it is medicine. By prioritizing whole, nutrient-dense foods and heart-healthy fats, individuals can profoundly influence their longevity, vitality, and quality of life. The Mediterranean diet isn't just a meal plan – it's a science-backed longevity blueprint. By embracing its rich variety of fruits, vegetables, whole grains, fish, and healthy fats, you can protect your heart, sharpen your mind, and extend your years with strength and vitality.

Caloric Restriction: Eating Less to Live Longer

Studies in animals and humans suggest that reducing calorie intake while maintaining proper nutrition can extend lifespan. The CALERIE Trial (Comprehensive Assessment of Long-term Effects of Reducing Intake of Energy) found that a 25 percent reduction in calorie intake improved metabolic markers and slowed aging.

The Okinawan Diet – rich in vegetables, soy, and small portions – has been linked to one of the highest concentrations of centenarians in the world. Mindful Eating Strategy: "Hara Hachi Bu," a Japanese principle meaning "Eat until you are 80 percent full," helps prevent overeating and promotes metabolic efficiency.

The Dangers of Processed Foods: The Silent Killer

Processed foods accelerate aging by increasing inflammation, damaging gut health, and promoting metabolic disorders. The three worst offenders are added sugars – cause insulin resistance and promote cellular aging; trans fats – increase heart disease risk and create oxidative stress; and preservatives and additives – disrupt the gut microbiome, weakening immunity.

Case Study: The Western Diet and Life Expectancy – A Recipe for Declining Health

In our modern world, convenience often trumps nutrition – but at what cost? The Western diet, dominated by processed foods, refined sugars, unhealthy fats, and excessive sodium, has become a leading driver of chronic disease and reduced life expectancy.

The Alarming Link Between Processed Foods and Chronic Illness, Obesity Epidemic

The Western diet is calorie-dense but nutrient-poor, filled with highly processed, sugary, and fried foods that promote weight gain, insulin resistance, and metabolic dysfunction. As a result, obesity rates have skyrocketed, increasing the risk of numerous life-threatening conditions. Diabetes on the Rise – diets heavy in refined carbohydrates and added sugars overwhelm the body's ability to regulate blood sugar, leading to insulin resistance, Type 2 diabetes, and widespread inflammation. Over time, this contributes to nerve damage, kidney disease, and cardiovascular complications. Cardiovascular Disease and Premature Aging – highly processed meats, trans fats, and excessive sodium in the Western diet clog arteries, raise blood pressure, and increase bad cholesterol (LDL), significantly elevating the risk of heart attacks and strokes. Studies show that countries adopting Western dietary patterns experience higher mortality rates from cardiovascular disease compared to those following traditional, whole-food-based diets. Reduced Life Expectancy – with its overwhelming contribution to chronic disease, systemic inflammation, and metabolic decline, the Western diet has been directly linked to shortened lifespan. Researchers have found that individuals consuming diets rich in ultra-processed foods have a significantly higher risk of premature death compared to those who prioritize whole, natural foods.

Science is clear: what we eat directly impacts how long and how well we live. The Western diet, though convenient, is fueling a public health crisis – one meal at a time. The Western diet is a fast track to chronic disease and reduced longevity. By moving away from processed foods and embracing whole, nutrient-dense meals, we can protect our bodies, extend our lives, and reclaim our health – one bite at a time. In contrast, populations that consume whole, minimally processed foods have lower rates of age-related diseases.

Implementing a Longevity Nutrition Plan

Aging gracefully isn't just about genetics – it's about deliberate choices, starting with what's on your plate. The foundation of any longevity-focused diet is whole, nutrient-dense foods that nourish the body at the cellular level, combat inflammation, and enhance vitality. By prioritizing clean, unprocessed ingredients, you're not just eating for today – you're investing in a longer, healthier future.

Prioritizing Whole Nutrient-Dense Foods.

The key to longevity lies in foods that come straight from nature, untainted by artificial additives and preservatives. Building your diet around vibrant fruits, fiber-rich vegetables, heart-healthy whole grains, nuts, and lean proteins ensures that your body receives a steady supply of antioxidants, essential vitamins, and minerals – all crucial for cellular repair and disease prevention. Fruits and vegetables: packed with polyphenols, fiber, and phytonutrients that reduce inflammation and oxidative stress. Whole grains: provide steady energy, gut-friendly fiber, and critical B vitamins for brain and metabolic health.

Nuts and seeds: rich in healthy fats, magnesium, and protein, supporting cardiovascular and cognitive function. Lean proteins (fish, legumes, pasture-raised poultry): build muscle, enhance recovery, and keep metabolism strong.

Ditch Ultra-Processed Foods and Opt for Homemade Alternatives

The fastest way to accelerate aging is through ultra-processed foods, laden with refined sugars, hydrogenated oils, artificial preservatives, and sodium. These foods contribute to chronic inflammation, insulin resistance, and metabolic disorders – all of which shorten lifespan. Instead, embrace homemade, whole-food-based meals that allow you to control ingredients, maximize nutrient density, and eliminate harmful additives. Avoid: packaged snacks, sugary sodas, flavored yogurts, instant oatmeal, fast food, frozen dinners, and processed meats. Replace with: freshly prepared meals using whole organic ingredients, infused with flavorful herbs and spices that enhance both taste and longevity.

Longevity starts in the kitchen. By prioritizing whole, nutrient-rich foods and eliminating ultra-processed meals, you're giving your body the tools it needs to thrive, repair, and resist the diseases of aging – one nourishing meal at a time.

Eating for Gut Health: Nourishing Your Microbiome for Longevity

Your gut isn't just responsible for digestion – it's often called "the second brain" because of its profound influence on immune function, mood regulation, metabolism, and even longevity. A thriving gut microbiome – filled with diverse, beneficial bacteria – is one of the most powerful tools for slowing aging, reducing inflammation, and enhancing overall vitality.

The Essentials of a Gut-Healthy Diet include Fermented Foods: The Probiotics Powerhouse

Fermented foods are nature's probiotics, teeming with live, beneficial bacteria that enhance digestion, strengthen immunity, and support mental clarity. These foods increase microbial diversity in the gut, helping to regulate metabolism and reduce the risk of chronic diseases like obesity, diabetes, and neurodegenerative conditions.

The Best Fermented Foods for Gut Health and Longevity are Kimchi and Sauerkraut – Kimchi and sauerkraut are two of the most effective fermented foods for supporting gut health and promoting longevity. Both are rich in probiotics – beneficial bacteria that help balance your gut microbiome, which plays a crucial role in digestion, immunity, mood regulation, and even inflammation control. Made from cabbage and other vegetables, these foods are also high in fiber and antioxidants. Their fermentation process produces powerful compounds that nourish the gut lining and enhance nutrient absorption. Regularly eating small servings of kimchi or sauerkraut can help improve digestive health, support immune function, and reduce age-related decline from the inside out.

Rich in probiotics and antioxidants that support immune resilience. Yogurt and Kefir – Packed with live cultures that improve digestion and gut barrier integrity.

Kombucha and Miso – Loaded with gut-friendly bacteria that aid in detoxification and inflammation control.

Prebiotic Fibers: Feeding Your Gut Microbiome. Probiotics thrive on prebiotic fibers, which act as fuel for beneficial gut bacteria, encouraging their growth and activity. By incorporating fiber-rich prebiotics into your diet, you're fortifying your microbiome, supporting digestion, and enhancing nutrient absorption.

Some of my favorites Top Prebiotic Foods to Strengthen Gut Bacteria include onions and garlic – contain natural antimicrobial and prebiotic compounds that balance gut flora. Asparagus and Leeks – High in inulin, a prebiotic fiber that fuels beneficial bacteria. Green Bananas and Oats – Provide resistant starches that nourish the gut microbiome and promote metabolic health. A healthy gut is the foundation of a long, vibrant life. By incorporating fermented foods and prebiotic-rich ingredients into your daily diet, you're actively feeding and fortifying your microbiome – enhancing digestion, boosting immunity, and unlocking the key to lasting wellness and longevity.

Personalized Nutrition: The Future of Longevity and Optimal Health

Gone are the days of one-size-fits-all diets. Science has now revealed that nutrition is deeply personal, and what works for one person may not work for another. The key to longevity lies in understanding your body's unique genetic makeup, metabolism, and microbiome – allowing you to fuel yourself in the most efficient and health-boosting way possible.

The Cutting-Edge Science of Personalized Nutrition. DNA-Based Testing: Unlocking Your Genetic Blueprint. Your DNA holds the key to your nutritional needs. Advanced testing services like Viome, 23andMe, and InsideTracker analyze genetic markers related to metabolism, nutrient absorption, and food sensitivities. This allows individuals to tailor their diets to their genetic strengths and weaknesses, optimizing nutrient intake for disease prevention, energy, and longevity.

DNA Testing Helps Personalize Diets

Determines how efficiently your body metabolizes fats, carbs, and proteins. Identifies genetic predispositions to deficiencies (e.g., vitamin D, B12, omega-3s). Pinpoints potential food sensitivities and inflammation triggers and customizes diet plans to reduce disease risk and enhance overall wellness. While these tools aren't perfect, they can provide helpful insights for tailoring your nutrition.

Microbiome Analysis: Fueling Your Gut for Longevity

Your gut microbiome is as unique as a fingerprint — and its health is directly tied to digestion, immune function, weight management, and even mental clarity. Microbiome testing services can analyze the composition of gut bacteria, helping individuals determine which foods promote balance, improve digestion, and prevent inflammation-related diseases. Microbiome Analysis Improves Health. Microbiome analysis identifies which foods enhance beneficial bacteria and which harm them. Helps optimize digestion and nutrient absorption. Reduces inflammation and improves immune function and customizes dietary recommendations for gut health, metabolism, and longevity. Personalized nutrition is the future of longevity. By using DNA-based testing and microbiome analysis, we can move beyond generic diet trends and create highly customized, precision-driven nutrition plans that optimize health, prevent disease, and unlock the body's full potential for a longer, healthier life.

Food as Fuel for a Vibrant Future

The journey to longevity starts on the plate. By making small, intentional dietary changes, we can boost energy levels, reduce inflammation, improve cognitive function, and extend our health span. Aging is inevitable – but how we age is a choice. When we treat food as medicine, we unlock the potential for a longer, healthier, more vibrant life.

You have just discovered how powerful food can be in rewriting your aging story – from reducing inflammation and boosting energy to rekindling joy and presence in everyday life. These changes may seem small, but they create a ripple effect that can transform how you live and feel. So, take a moment to celebrate – you have taken a meaningful step toward a stronger, more vibrant you. "What will you try first? Next, we'll build on this foundation with movement and exercise – another essential key to feeling youthful, capable, and fully engaged in life. Keep going – you're doing great, and your next chapter is already in motion.

CHAPTER 4:
THE WEIGHT OF TIME
AND LONELINESS

"Motion is medicine. Move your body,
and your body will move you forward."
— Maria L. Ellis, BBA, MBA

I met Evelyn at a vulnerable moment – standing at the edge of her driveway, unsure if she could make it to the mailbox without losing her breath. At seventy-two, she found herself growing weaker, more fatigued, and increasingly dependent on others for simple tasks. She longed to keep up with her grandchildren, to tend her beloved garden without pain, and to reclaim the independence that seemed to be slipping away. In this chapter, you'll meet Evelyn, whose story shows how small, consistent steps can lead to meaningful change. She didn't start with a gym membership or a personal trainer – just daily walks around the block and light stretching in her living room. Through her journey, we'll break down the science of strength training, cardio, balance, and flexibility in simple terms. You'll see that building a more active, energized body isn't about doing everything at once – it's about doing what you can, where you are, and knowing it's never too late to begin.

Strength training became Evelyn's first milestone. In

the beginning, even wall push-ups felt impossible, and lifting light hand weights made her arms tremble. But slowly, patiently, her body adapted. Weeks into her new routine, Evelyn beamed with pride as she completed her first full push-up on the floor – a small but powerful victory that reawakened her sense of self. Cardio followed a similar path.

Yet day after day, she pushed a little further, and the day she completed an uninterrupted fifteen-minute walk around her neighborhood felt like winning a marathon. Balance and flexibility training brought even more confidence. Standing on one foot without wobbling, stretching down to touch her toes – these achievements, once unthinkable, opened new doors to independence and joy. Evelyn's story reminds us that progress is not linear. There were setbacks – days of soreness, doubt, and weather that kept her indoors. But consistency, not perfection, carried her forward. Today, Evelyn plays tag with her grandkids, travels with ease, and gardens for hours, living proof that movement is the medicine for a longer, fuller life.

As you move through this chapter, I invite you to see Evelyn not as an exception, but as a reflection of what's possible for all of us. Whether you're just starting out or looking to deepen your commitment, transformation begins with one small, intentional step. For Evelyn, it was placing a yoga mat beside her bed and doing two gentle stretches each morning before reaching for her phone. For you, it might be a five-minute walk after lunch, filling a water bottle each morning, or simply standing up and moving during commercial breaks. Whatever it is, let it be simple, doable, and a loving reminder that you're choosing to care for yourself – one step at a time.

Evelyn didn't become a marathon runner or join a boot camp. She simply reclaimed her body, one movement at a time. And that's exactly what this chapter is about – rediscovering your vitality not through punishment or perfection, but through joyful, sustainable motion that supports the life you want to live. In the quest for a longer, healthier life, exercise is not optional – it is essential.

Physical activity is a cornerstone of longevity, influencing every system in the body, from cardiovascular health to brain function and even cellular repair. Many of us have been conditioned to think of exercise as something we do to lose weight or build muscle, but its role in longevity is much deeper. Movement is the ultimate form of medicine, capable of reversing aging at a cellular level, increasing energy, improving mental clarity, and preserving our independence well into old age.

As we grow older, staying active becomes even more critical. The body thrives on movement. Those who incorporate regular exercise into their daily routine enjoy stronger bones, healthier hearts, sharper minds, and increased resilience to disease. In contrast, a sedentary lifestyle accelerates aging, leading to muscle loss, chronic pain, cognitive decline, and diminished quality of life.

This chapter will explore how exercise influences longevity, the types of movement that provide the most benefit, and practical ways to incorporate fitness into daily life – regardless of age or ability.

The Science of Exercise and Longevity

Exercise is one of the few scientifically proven ways to slow down the aging process. It works at the cellular level, triggering a cascade of biological processes that protect against disease, boost energy, and improve overall health.

Boosting Mitochondrial Health: Energizing Your Cells for Longevity

At the core of every cell lie the mitochondria. These microscopic energy generators are responsible for producing adenosine triphosphate (ATP), the fuel that powers every heartbeat, thought, and movement. Without healthy mitochondria, the body's ability to function at its peak is compromised, leading to fatigue, muscle weakness, cognitive decline, and a sluggish metabolism.

As we age, mitochondrial efficiency naturally declines, reducing energy production and accelerating cellular aging. This decline contributes to chronic fatigue, muscle loss, slower recovery, and an increased risk of age-related diseases. However, the good news is that mitochondria are highly adaptable, and with the right strategies, you can enhance their function, increase energy production, and slow the aging process.

By optimizing nutrition, engaging in mitochondrial-boosting exercise, and incorporating targeted longevity strategies, you can supercharge your energy levels, sharpen cognitive function, and maintain a vibrant, youthful body well into your later years. Your mitochondria hold the key to sustained energy and longevity. Nurturing them through proper diet, movement, and lifestyle habits will not only help you combat fatigue but also unlock greater vitality, resilience, and extended health span.

Regular aerobic exercise – such as brisk walking, swimming, or cycling – stimulates mitochondrial biogenesis, the process of creating new mitochondria. This means more energy, increased endurance, and a stronger, more resilient body. High-Intensity Interval Training (HIIT), which involves short bursts of intense effort followed by rest, is particularly effective for improving mitochondrial health. Studies show that HIIT can enhance mitochondrial function in older adults, leading to better endurance and metabolic health. However, individuals with health conditions should consult a physician before starting high-intensity training.

Reducing Chronic Inflammation

Inflammation is a silent contributor to aging and a major driver of diseases like heart disease, diabetes, and neurodegenerative disorders. Exercise acts as a natural anti-inflammatory, reducing the production of harmful cytokines (inflammatory chemical messengers) while promoting anti-inflammatory molecules like interleukin-10. Additionally, exercise positively influences gut health, leading to a more diverse and balanced gut microbiome, which plays a crucial role in immune regulation and inflammation control. Interleukin-10 (IL-10) is a powerful anti-inflammatory cytokine that plays a critical role in modulating the immune system, preventing chronic inflammation, and promoting tissue repair. Often referred to as the "peacekeeper" of the immune response, IL-10 works by balancing pro-inflammatory signals, ensuring that the immune system responds effectively to threats without causing excessive damage to healthy tissues.

As we age, chronic low-grade inflammation – often called "inflammaging" – becomes a major driver of disease and cellular decline. Elevated inflammation contributes to neurodegeneration, cardiovascular disease, autoimmune disorders, and metabolic dysfunction. IL-10 acts as a counterbalance, reducing excessive inflammatory responses that accelerate aging.

Increasing Telomere Length: Slowing Cellular Aging

Deep within our cells lies a biological clock that dictates how we age – telomeres. These protective caps at the ends of our chromosomes shield our DNA from damage, much like the plastic tips on shoelaces prevent fraying. However, as we age, telomeres naturally shorten, leading to cellular aging, reduced regeneration, and an increased risk of chronic diseases like heart disease, neurodegeneration, and cancer.

But here's the exciting part: Telomere shortening isn't inevitable. Science has revealed that lifestyle choices – especially physical activity – can slow, and even reverse, telomere attrition, effectively extending cellular health and longevity.

Physical Activity and Telomere Length – Studies have shown that regular exercise is directly linked to longer telomeres, meaning that movement isn't just good for muscles – it slows aging at the DNA level. People who maintain an active lifestyle tend to have biologically younger cells, offering protection against age-related decline. Endurance Training and Telomerase Activation – Engaging in aerobic and endurance-based activities – such as running, cycling, swimming, and brisk walking – stimulates telomerase, the enzyme responsible for maintaining and rebuilding telomeres. This means that every workout strengthens your body and activates your cellular repair system, helping your DNA resist aging. Cellular Renewal and Longevity – Exercise also reduces oxidative stress and inflammation, two major contributors to telomere shortening. By staying active, you're shielding your cells from damage, enhancing repair mechanisms, and optimizing longevity at the most fundamental level.

Your lifestyle choices directly influence how fast or slow your cells age. By incorporating regular endurance exercise, you can activate telomerase, preserve telomere length, and extend the health and lifespan of your cells – unlocking a longer, stronger, and more youthful life from the inside out.

Enhancing Cardiovascular Health: Strengthening Your Heart for Longevity

Your heart is more than just an organ – it's the engine that powers your body, pumping life-sustaining oxygen and nutrients to every cell. Just like any other muscle, it requires consistent exercise to stay strong, efficient, and resilient against the effects of aging. Neglecting cardiovascular health increases the risk of hypertension, heart disease, and stroke, while prioritizing heart-friendly activities enhances circulation, boosts energy, and extends lifespan.

The life-changing benefits of cardiovascular exercise lower blood pressure – Regular movement strengthens the heart muscle, allowing it to pump blood more efficiently, reducing strain on the arteries and lowering blood pressure naturally. Improves blood circulation – A strong heart enhances oxygen and nutrient delivery to the brain, muscles, and organs, boosting cognitive function, endurance, and overall vitality. Balances cholesterol levels – Cardiovascular activity helps reduce harmful LDL cholesterol, which clogs arteries, while simultaneously increasing beneficial HDL cholesterol, which clears fatty deposits, keeping the heart and blood vessels in peak condition. Promotes new blood vessel growth (angiogenesis) – Exercise stimulates the formation of new blood vessels, ensuring greater oxygen supply to tissues and improving overall cardiovascular efficiency.

You don't need a gym membership to improve your heart health. Simple, enjoyable activities can have dramatic effects on cardiovascular function and longevity: Walking – A low-impact, highly effective way to strengthen the heart, improve circulation, and enhance endurance. Swimming – A full-body workout that boosts heart health while being easy on the joints, making it an excellent choice for all ages. Dancing – I love to dance; it elevates the heart rate while reducing stress and improving coordination, making it one of the most fun ways to enhance cardiovascular function. A strong heart is a long-life heart. By incorporating heart-healthy exercises into your daily routine, you can improve circulation, lower disease risk, and boost overall vitality – ensuring a healthier, longer life filled with energy and strength.

Enhancing Brain Function and Preventing Cognitive Decline: The Power of Movement for a Sharper Mind

Exercise isn't just a workout for your body – it's vital fuel for your brain. Just as physical activity strengthens muscles and improves circulation, it nourishes and protects the brain, enhancing mental clarity, memory, and cognitive resilience.

Every time you move, your heart pumps oxygen-rich

blood to the brain, delivering essential nutrients that fuel neurons, repair cellular damage, and support optimal cognitive function. Increased circulation also flushes out toxins and reduces oxidative stress, two key factors in neurodegeneration. Activating Brain-Derived Neurotrophic Factor (BDNF) – often called "Miracle-Gro for the brain," BDNF is a powerful protein released during exercise that stimulates the growth of new neurons, strengthens neural pathways, and enhances brain plasticity. Higher BDNF levels are directly linked to a reduced risk of Alzheimer's, Parkinson's, and other neurodegenerative diseases – essentially helping the brain stay sharp and adaptive well into old age. Movement + Mental Stimulation = Maximum Brain Benefits – certain physical activities provide an extra cognitive boost by engaging both body and mind simultaneously. Activities like dance classes, martial arts, and even sports that require strategy and coordination challenge the brain to process information quickly, improve memory retention, and enhance problem-solving skills – acting as a double defense against cognitive decline. Your brain thrives on movement. By staying active and engaging in activities that challenge both the body and mind, you can increase BDNF, enhance cognitive function, and safeguard against memory loss – ensuring a sharp, resilient brain for years to come.

Strength Training: The Ultimate Key to Aging Strong and Gracefully

Aging isn't just about growing older – it's about maintaining strength, vitality, and independence. One of the greatest threats to longevity is sarcopenia, the gradual loss of muscle mass that occurs with age. Left unchecked, sarcopenia leads to weakness, frailty, poor balance, and an increased risk of falls and fractures. But there's a proven way to combat it: strength training.

Also known as resistance training, strength training isn't just for athletes – it's a lifelong investment in your body's ability to move, function, and thrive. By incorporating regular strength-building exercises, you can maintain lean muscle, protect your bones, and enhance your overall health well into your later years.

The Power of Strength Training for Longevity

Preserves Muscle Mass and Prevents Sarcopenia – strength training helps counteract age-related muscle loss, keeping the body strong, stable, and capable of everyday movements. Builds Bone Density and Prevents Osteoporosis – resistance exercises increase bone mineral density, reducing the risk of fractures and protecting against osteoporosis – a major concern for aging adults. Improves Posture and Joint Stability – strengthening the muscles that support your spine and joints reduces strain, alleviates pain, and enhances mobility, making daily activities easier and more comfortable.

Boosts Metabolism and Supports Healthy Weight – lean muscle is metabolically active, meaning the more muscle you have, the more calories you burn – even at rest. Strength training helps maintain a healthy weight and reduces fat accumulation, particularly around the abdomen. Reduces the Risk of Falls and Injuries – strong muscles enhance balance, coordination, and reaction time, significantly lowering the risk of falls, fractures, and long-term immobility.

Strength training isn't just about fitness – it's about aging with confidence, resilience, and independence. By incorporating regular resistance exercises, you can preserve muscle, strengthen bones, and enhance mobility – ensuring you stay active, agile, and empowered for years to come.

Strength Training Exercises for Longevity: Build Strength, Stability, and Resilience

Strength training isn't just about building muscle – it's about future-proofing your body for a long, healthy, and active life. The right exercises help maintain mobility, prevent injuries, and preserve independence well into old age. By incorporating these fundamental movements into your routine, you'll enhance muscle strength, improve posture, and keep your joints strong and pain-free.

The following are essential strength training movements for lifelong vitality:

- Squats – The Ultimate Longevity Move. Why? Squats are a full-body powerhouse exercise that strengthens the legs, glutes, and core, helping to maintain balance, mobility, and functional strength for everyday movements like standing, climbing stairs, and getting up from a chair. Squats improve leg endurance, joint stability, and bone density, reducing the risk of falls and fractures.
- Lunges – Balance and Lower Body Power. Why? Lunges challenge coordination and stability while strengthening the quads, hamstrings, and glutes. They improve single-leg strength, which is essential for maintaining agility and preventing falls. Lunges enhance core control, balance, and lower body strength, promoting smooth, pain-free movement.
- Push-ups – A Full-Body Upper Strength Booster. Why? Push-ups build upper body and core strength, working the chest, shoulders, arms, and abs. This classic move is key to maintaining the strength needed for daily tasks like lifting, pushing, and carrying objects.
- Push-ups help prevent age-related muscle loss in the upper body, keeping the shoulders and arms strong and mobile.
- Bent-over Rows – Strengthen Your Back and Improve Posture. Why? Bent-over rows target the upper and mid-back muscles, improving posture and spinal alignment. A strong back reduces the risk of slouching, chronic pain, and spinal degradation over time. Promote a strong, upright pos-

ture, reduce back pain, and protect against age-related spinal weakness.

- Planks – Core Stability for a Pain-Free Back. Why? Planks are a powerful core stabilizer, strengthening the abs, lower back, and deep core muscles that protect the spine. A strong core is essential for balance, posture, and injury prevention. Planks help reduce back pain, improve flexibility, and support healthy movement patterns as you age.

Longevity isn't just about living longer – it's about staying strong, mobile, and independent as you age. Incorporating these foundational strength exercises into your routine will enhance endurance, protect against injuries, and keep your body resilient for decades to come.

Case Study: The Pvolve Program and Menopausal Women – Unlocking Strength, Flexibility, and Vitality

Menopause is often associated with muscle loss, joint stiffness, and decreased mobility, but what if the right exercise program could reverse these effects and restore strength, flexibility, and confidence?

A groundbreaking study examined the impact of low-impact resistance training through the Pvolve Program on women aged forty to sixty, a demographic often overlooked in fitness research. The results were astonishing: participants increased lower body strength by 20 percent, improving stability, balance, and the ability to perform daily activities with ease. Flexibility improved by 21 percent, reducing stiffness, enhancing mobility, and preventing the joint pain commonly associated with menopause.

What made Pvolve's method unique was its focus on functional, controlled movements, targeting muscle activation without excessive strain on the joints. Unlike high-impact workouts that can lead to injuries, this program offered a sustainable, body-friendly approach – allowing women to rebuild strength and flexibility without risking overuse injuries.

Women in the study reported feeling more agile, energized, and empowered, proving that menopause is not a decline but an opportunity to build a stronger, more resilient body.

Low-impact resistance training isn't just about fitness – it's a gateway to longevity, independence, and pain-free movement. By incorporating targeted strength and flexibility exercises, menopausal women can transform their bodies, boost mobility, and regain the confidence to move with ease at any age.

Case Study: Kettlebell Training for Older Adults – Building Strength, Resilience, and Longevity

Aging does not mean losing strength – it means finding smarter ways to maintain and enhance it. A year-long study explored the transformative effects of kettlebell training on adults aged sixty to eighty, revealing remarkable improvements in muscle mass, grip strength, and inflammation reduction.

Participants saw notable gains in lean muscle, counteracting the natural decline caused by aging (sarcopenia). Maintaining muscle mass is crucial for mobility, balance, and overall independence. Enhanced Grip Strength – often overlooked, grip strength is a strong predictor of longevity and functional fitness. Kettlebell training improved participants' ability to carry, lift, and perform daily tasks with greater ease, reducing the risk of falls and injuries. Chronic inflammation is a silent driver of aging and disease. The study found that consistent kettlebell training lowered inflammatory markers, supporting joint health, cardiovascular function, and overall well-being.

What makes kettlebell training so effective for older adults is its combination of strength, stability, and endurance training in one dynamic movement. Unlike traditional weightlifting, kettlebell workouts engage multiple muscle groups, improve coordination, and enhance functional movement patterns, making everyday activities easier and safer.

Participants in the study reported feeling stronger, more confident, and more capable in their daily lives – proving that it's never too late to rebuild strength and vitality. Kettlebell training isn't just about fitness – it's about reclaiming strength, resilience, and independence as you age. With simple, functional movements, older adults can enhance muscle mass, boost grip strength, and fight inflammation – ensuring a longer, healthier, and more active life.

Essential Flexibility and Balance Training for Longevity

Yoga and Tai Chi – I practice yoga for mastering control and coordination. Gentle yet powerful, these ancient practices are scientifically proven to enhance flexibility, balance, and coordination. Yoga elongates muscles and improves range of motion, while Tai Chi strengthens stabilizing muscles and enhances mind-body awareness – a key component in preventing stumbles and missteps.

Single-Leg Stands – Stability for Everyday Movements. Simple but effective, standing on one leg for thirty seconds at a time strengthens ankles, knees, and hip stabilizers, reinforcing the core and postural muscles needed for steady, controlled movement. This drill mimics real-life balance challenges, reducing the risk of unexpected falls.

Hand-Eye Coordination Drills – Keeping Reflexes Sharp. Balance isn't just about lower-body strength – it's about reaction time and spatial awareness. Activities like catching a ball, tossing a beanbag, or practicing quick hand movements stimulate neural pathways, improving reflexes, agility, and coordination – ensuring the body responds instinctively and effectively to sudden movements or obstacles.

Balance and flexibility are the foundation of lifelong

mobility. By incorporating targeted training, you can strengthen stabilizing muscles, improve reflexes, and enhance flexibility – ensuring you move with confidence, prevent falls, and enjoy an active, independent life well into old age.

Movement Is Medicine – The Key to Aging Strong

Aging isn't about slowing down – it's about adapting, strengthening, and staying active with purpose. Every step, stretch, and rep we take is an investment in our longevity, independence, and vitality.

To live longer, feel stronger, and thrive at every stage of life, we must commit to a movement-rich lifestyle that supports total-body wellness including Strength Training – To preserve muscle mass, prevent frailty, and maintain power. Cardiovascular Exercise – To keep the heart strong, boost circulation, and energize the body. Flexibility and Balance Training – To enhance mobility, reduce stiffness, and prevent falls. Daily Movement – Because motion is medicine, and an active body is a thriving body.

Our bodies were designed to move, and the more we move, the better we age. By embracing movement as a lifelong habit, not a chore, we ensure that our golden years are filled with strength, agility, and limitless potential. So where will you start? The secret to longevity isn't found in a pill – it's found in movement. Stay strong, stay active, and age with power, grace, and resilience.

CHAPTER 5:
THE HEALING POWER OF SLEEP: RESETTING YOUR BODY'S NATURAL RHYTHM

"A well-rested body is a well-repaired body.
Sleep is the foundation of renewal."
— Maria L. Ellis, BBA, MBA

Sleep is not a luxury; it's a biological necessity. In today's fast-paced world, many people treat sleep as optional, sacrificing hours of deep rest in favor of productivity or entertainment. Yet mounting research shows that sleep is one of the most powerful levers we have to extend our lifespan, protect our brain health, and regenerate every cell in our body. In this chapter, we'll explore the profound connection between sleep and longevity – and discover simple, effective ways to realign our natural rhythms for healing, energy, and vibrant living. By the end, you'll see sleep not just as a nightly obligation, but as a powerful act of self-preservation and vitality.

Ever woken up feeling like you aged ten years overnight? Puffy eyes, dull skin, heavy limbs, you wonder, What happened? That's how crucial sleep can be. It's not just about feeling rested; it's about protecting your brain, your body, and your spirit from the wear and tear of time.

When sleep slips, everything else does too – your memory, your mood, your metabolism, your ability to show up fully in life.

If you want to stay sharp, strong, and emotionally present, sleep is non-negotiable. Sleep is where the body repairs, the mind resets, and cellular aging slows. Without it, even the best diet and exercise plan won't get you far. But here's the good news: this chapter isn't about shaming you for your restless nights. It's about helping you reclaim them – so you can wake up feeling clear, strong, and younger. Yes, younger. Because sleep is the most natural, powerful longevity tool you already have.

Quality sleep does more than clear your head – it actively extends your health span, the number of years you live with strength, clarity, and independence. When you sleep deeply and consistently, your body repairs damaged cells, balances hormones, and clears the brain of toxins linked to cognitive decline. But just as important, sleep restores your emotional resilience. It lifts the fog that can leave you feeling detached, irritable, or withdrawn. Think back to Sofia – sitting by the window, feeling disconnected and adrift. Poor sleep can quietly pull us into that same state of loneliness and confusion. But great sleep? It brings us back. It sharpens the mind, lightens the mood, and fuels the energy we need to engage with life and the people we love.

Why Sleep is the Ultimate Longevity Tool

In the quest for a longer, healthier life, sleep is often overlooked. While we focus on nutrition and exercise, sleep remains the silent pillar of longevity, playing a crucial role in cellular repair, immune function, and cognitive health.

Sleep is not simply a time of rest – it is an active, dynamic process where the body and mind undergo critical recovery and rejuvenation. During deep sleep, our cells repair damage, our brain detoxifies itself, and our metabolism resets. Yet, modern life often sacrifices sleep for productivity, entertainment, and digital distractions. The result? Chronic sleep deprivation, which accelerates aging, weakens the immune system, and increases the risk of disease.

This chapter will explore the profound connection between sleep and longevity, examining the biological mechanisms at play and providing science-backed strategies to improve sleep quality for a longer, healthier life.

The Science of Sleep and Longevity

Sleep is a biological necessity, influencing everything from cellular repair to brain function. It is divided into several stages, each with distinct roles in recovery and renewal. Understanding these stages helps us appreciate why deep, uninterrupted sleep is essential for health and longevity.

Cellular Detoxification: The Brain's Nightly Cleanup

One of the most important functions of sleep is detoxification, particularly in the brain. During deep sleep, the glymphatic system (the brain's waste clearance system) becomes highly active. It flushes out toxins, metabolic waste, and harmful proteins like amyloid-beta, which have been linked to Alzheimer's disease.

A groundbreaking study published in Science found that this process is ten times more active during sleep than wakefulness, highlighting why poor sleep increases the risk of neurodegenerative diseases. Prioritizing deep sleep reduces the buildup of toxic waste in the brain and protects against cognitive decline.

Hormonal Regulation: The Sleep-Hormone Connection

Sleep is a fundamental pillar of health, playing a crucial role in balancing essential hormones that regulate metabolism, stress response, and overall well-being. During deep sleep, growth hormone is released, facilitating tissue repair, muscle growth, and bone density maintenance, ensuring the body's regenerative processes function optimally. At the same time, melatonin, often referred to as the "sleep hormone," governs the circadian rhythm, promoting restful sleep while also acting as a potent antioxidant that combats cellular aging. Meanwhile, cortisol, the body's primary stress hormone, naturally declines at night, allowing for deep recovery and restoration. However, chronic sleep deprivation disrupts this delicate hormonal balance, leading to elevated stress levels, weight gain, metabolic dysfunction, and an increased risk of age-related diseases. Quality sleep is not just about rest – it is essential for hormonal balance, longevity, and disease prevention, reinforcing the need for consistent, restorative sleep habits.

DNA Repair: The Secret to Slowing Down Aging

Every day, our cells endure relentless assaults – from environmental pollutants, harmful toxins, and the very metabolic processes that sustain life. Yet, nature has equipped us with an extraordinary defense system: DNA repair mechanisms that work tirelessly to undo this daily damage. And when do these microscopic repair teams operate at their peak? During sleep – the body's most powerful regeneration phase.

One of the most vital factors in cellular aging is telomere length – the protective caps at the ends of our chromosomes that act as biological clocks. Telomeres prevent our DNA from fraying. However, as we age, these caps naturally shorten, accelerating cellular deterioration and increasing the risk of chronic disease.

Groundbreaking research published in Sleep reveals a fascinating connection: individuals who consistently get high-quality rest tend to have longer telomeres. This suggests that sleep isn't just about feeling rested – it's a fundamental pillar of longevity, preserving DNA integrity and slowing cellular aging. Prioritizing deep, restorative sleep isn't just a luxury – it's a science-backed strategy to protect your cells, extend your lifespan, and unlock the secrets of graceful aging.

The Consequences of Sleep Deprivation

Few lifestyle habits are as detrimental to longevity as chronic sleep deprivation. Skimping on rest doesn't just leave you groggy – it accelerates biological aging, weakens vital systems, and dramatically increases the risk of life-threatening diseases. Sleep isn't a passive state; it's a critical period for cellular repair, hormone regulation, and brain detoxification. When we neglect it, our health pays the price.

The Health Risks of Poor Sleep include Cardiovascular Disease

Insufficient sleep triggers a dangerous rise in blood pressure, fuels inflammation, and significantly increases the risk of heart attacks, strokes, and arterial damage. Metabolic Disorders – Sleep deprivation disrupts insulin sensitivity, leading to uncontrolled blood sugar spikes, increased fat storage, and a higher likelihood of obesity and type 2 diabetes. Cognitive Decline – A tired brain is a vulnerable brain. Chronic sleep loss impairs memory, focus, and critical thinking, while also heightening the risk of neurodegenerative diseases like Alzheimer's and Parkinson's. Immune System Suppression – Even a single night of poor sleep can weaken immune defenses, leaving you more prone to infections, chronic inflammation, and long-term disease.

Prioritizing deep, restorative sleep is just as vital as nutrition and exercise in safeguarding your health and extending your lifespan.

Stories like the case studies below – and perhaps even your own – show us that when sleep improves, everything improves. One woman I worked with had struggled with chronic insomnia for years. She believed her forgetfulness and low energy were just part of getting older. But once we addressed her sleep – establishing a calming evening routine, reducing caffeine, and creating a true rest environment – everything shifted. Her memory sharpened, her mood lifted, and she found herself laughing more, engaging more, living more. That's the true power of sleep. It's not just a passive state – it's one of your most active defenses against accelerated aging, mental decline, and emotional disconnection. If we want to age well, we have to sleep well. It's that simple.

The Whitehall II Study: The Deadly Cost of Sleep Deprivation

This study hits closer to home than most realize; researchers followed thousands of British civil servants through their daily routines, stress, and sleep habits. Known as the Whitehall II Study, it uncovered something striking: consistently losing just two hours of sleep each night didn't just lead to fatigue – it significantly increased the risk of chronic illness and early death. This wasn't about extreme deprivation, but the kind of quiet sleep loss many of us accept as normal – staying up late to catch up on work, scrolling through our phones, or watching just one more episode. The study's findings were clear: when sleep suffers, so does your long-term health.

For years, these dedicated professionals sacrificed sleep in the name of productivity, whittling their nightly rest from a healthy seven hours to a mere five. They pushed through exhaustion, fueled by caffeine and a relentless work ethic, believing that a few hours less sleep wouldn't matter. But science proved otherwise.

The study's findings were shocking and undeniable – those who consistently slept only five hours per night had double the risk of mortality, particularly from cardiovascular disease. Their hearts bore the brunt of chronic sleep deprivation, enduring higher blood pressure, increased inflammation, and a heightened risk of fatal heart attacks and strokes. The very drive that propelled them forward was, paradoxically, pulling them toward an early grave.

This research sent shockwaves through the medical and scientific communities, reinforcing what many had long suspected: sleep is not just a period of rest – it is a critical pillar of survival. Without it, the body deteriorates, the immune system weakens, and the heart suffers irreparable damage.

If you think sacrificing sleep for success is a worthy trade-off, think again. The price of chronic sleep deprivation isn't just exhaustion – it's an increased risk of premature death. Prioritizing at least seven hours of quality sleep each night isn't just an act of self-care; it's a life-saving decision.

The Telomere and Sleep Study

A study published in Sleep found that better sleep quality was directly linked to longer telomeres, protecting against cellular aging. In the realm of longevity science, one discovery stands out as a biological key to aging gracefully – telomeres. These tiny, protective caps at the ends of our chromosomes act like the plastic tips on shoelaces, preventing genetic unraveling. The longer they remain intact, the healthier and more youthful our cells stay.

But what if the secret to preserving these cellular guardians isn't found in an expensive serum or a cutting-edge drug, but rather in something far more accessible – sleep?

A groundbreaking study published in the journal Sleep uncovered a remarkable link between sleep quality and telomere length. Researchers found that individuals who consistently enjoyed deep, high-quality sleep had significantly longer telomeres, while those who suffered from fragmented, insufficient rest showed signs of accelerated cellular aging.

The implications were profound: better sleep doesn't

just help you feel refreshed – it actively slows down the biological clock, protecting against premature aging and age-related diseases. Every night of deep, uninterrupted sleep serves as a repair cycle for your DNA, safeguarding your cells from decline.

This research solidified what sleep scientists had long suspected: sleep isn't just about energy restoration – it's a powerful, natural defense against aging itself. A good night's sleep is more than just rest – it's an anti-aging elixir. By prioritizing consistent, high-quality sleep, you're not just improving your daily well-being – you're preserving your telomeres, protecting your DNA, and extending your health span.

The Cognitive Impact of Sleep Deprivation: A Silent Thief of Mental Clarity

In the relentless pursuit of success, many sacrifice sleep, believing they can push through fatigue with sheer determination. But what if every restless night wasn't just costing you energy – but erasing pieces of your mind?

A sobering report published in The International Journal of Environmental Research unveiled a chilling truth: chronic sleep deprivation leads to irreversible cognitive decline over time. Unlike short-term fatigue that can be reversed with a good night's rest, the long-term impact of persistent sleep loss is far more insidious – it chips away at memory, dulls cognitive sharpness, and accelerates brain aging.

The study's findings echoed a growing body of research: when sleep is sacrificed, so is brain health. The brain relies on deep sleep to clear out toxic waste, consolidate memories, and regenerate neural pathways. Without it, plaques associated with neurodegenerative diseases like Alzheimer's build up, neurons become damaged, and cognitive function steadily deteriorates.

For those who believe they can "catch up" on sleep later, science warns otherwise. The damage from chronic deprivation is often permanent, leaving individuals more vulnerable to dementia, forgetfulness, and mental fog that no amount of caffeine can fix.

Sleep isn't just a break from the day – it's a lifeline for cognitive longevity. Protecting your brain starts with prioritizing consistent, high-quality sleep, ensuring a sharper mind, better memory, and a future free from premature cognitive decline.

Creating the Perfect Sleep Environment

Optimizing your sleep environment is essential for deep, restorative sleep.

Bedroom Optimization

Your bedroom isn't just a place to sleep – it's a haven for healing, rejuvenation, and longevity. The quality of your sleep is directly influenced by your surroundings, and by fine-tuning your sleep environment, you can unlock deeper, more restorative rest that enhances brain function, immune strength, and overall well-being.

Bedroom Optimization: Transform Your Space into a Sleep Oasis. Keep it Cool – Your body naturally lowers its core temperature during sleep. Set your bedroom between 60 to 67°F to signal your brain that it's time to rest, promoting faster sleep onset and deeper sleep cycles. Eliminate Light – Even the smallest sliver of light can disrupt melatonin production, the hormone that regulates sleep. Use blackout curtains, an eye mask, or dim red nightlights to create a pitch-black environment that maximizes melatonin release.

Reduce Noise – Sudden sounds can jolt you out of deep sleep, even if you don't fully wake up. White noise machines, soft earplugs, or calming nature sounds can help drown out disruptions, keeping you in restorative sleep for longer. Invest in Quality Bedding – Your bed should be an inviting retreat, not a source of discomfort. Upgrade to a supportive mattress and pillows suited to your sleep position, and choose breathable, luxurious bedding that cradles you into blissful slumber. Creating the perfect sleep environment is one of the most powerful, science-backed ways to enhance your health and longevity. By cooling your room, eliminating light, reducing noise, and upgrading your bedding, you can unlock deep, uninterrupted sleep that restores your mind and body – every single night.

Mastering Light Exposure: Aligning Your Body with Nature's Rhythms

Light is one of the most powerful regulators of your body's internal clock, influencing everything from energy levels to sleep quality. By harnessing the right light at the right time, you can optimize your circadian rhythm, enhance melatonin production, and unlock deeper, more restorative sleep.

Morning Light: Set the Tone for the Day. Bask in Natural Sunlight Within Thirty Minutes of Waking – Stepping outside and exposing your eyes to natural sunlight first thing in the morning signals to your brain that it's time to wake up, suppressing melatonin and increasing alertness. Aim for ten to thirty minutes of sunlight exposure (even on cloudy days) to regulate your circadian rhythm and boost mood-enhancing serotonin levels.

Evening Light: Prepare Your Body for Rest. Reduce Blue Light Exposure at Night – Artificial blue light from phones, tablets, and LED screens tricks your brain into thinking it's still daytime, delaying melatonin production and making it harder to fall asleep. Dim the lights, switch to warm lighting, and power down screens at least one to two hours before bed. If screen time is unavoidable, wear blue-light blocking glasses or use screen filters to minimize disruption. Light is a powerful sleep regulator. By embracing morning sunlight to energize your day and reducing blue light exposure in the evening, you can synchronize your body's natural rhythms, improve sleep quality, and enhance overall well-being.

Sleep is not merely the absence of wakefulness; it is an active, vital process where your body repairs, your brain reorganizes, and your spirit renews. When you honor your circadian rhythm and cultivate a restful evening routine, you invest in one of the most powerful longevity tools available to you. True healing begins in the quiet moments when you allow your body the time and space it needs to restore itself. As we turn the page to the next chapter, we'll explore how mastering stress and recovery builds upon this foundation, empowering you to move through life's demands with greater resilience, strength, and ease.

CHAPTER 6:
MASTERING STRESS AND RECOVERY: BUILDING RESILIENCE FOR A LONGER LIFE

Just as sleep restores and renews us during the night, learning to manage stress and embrace recovery allows us to protect and strengthen our health throughout the day. In our modern world, stress has become an inescapable part of daily life, but it doesn't have to be destructive. When we understand how to work with our body's natural recovery systems, we can transform stress from a silent saboteur into a powerful teacher. In this chapter, we'll explore how chronic stress impacts the aging process, why intentional recovery is essential for longevity, and how you can build simple daily habits that promote resilience, balance, and emotional well-being.

Advanced Tools for Deeper Rest and Recovery

As science delves deeper into the mysteries of sleep, groundbreaking innovations are emerging to supercharge recovery, enhance sleep quality, and optimize brain function. These cutting-edge sleep technologies are rewriting the rules of rest, offering powerful tools to improve relaxation, reduce inflammation, and align the body's natural rhythms.

Game-Changing Sleep and Recovery Innovations

BrainTap. Brain Fitness App – Unlock the power of guided meditation, neuro-synchronization, and binaural beats to rewire your brain for better sleep. I enjoy this innovative application; it uses sound frequencies to shift brainwave activity, helping you de-stress, enhance focus, and enter deeper states of rest and recovery.

Hyperbaric Oxygen Therapy (HBOT) – Step into the future of cellular rejuvenation. HBOT floods the bloodstream with pure oxygen, promoting faster recovery, reducing inflammation, and enhancing brain function. This therapy is gaining traction as a powerful longevity tool, accelerating healing and boosting sleep efficiency by reducing oxidative stress.

Weighted Blankets – Experience the soothing embrace of deep pressure stimulation (DPS). Weighted blankets have been scientifically proven to reduce cortisol (the stress hormone), boost serotonin, and increase melatonin production, helping you fall asleep faster and stay asleep longer. The gentle, grounding pressure calms the nervous system, making it an excellent solution for those struggling with anxiety and insomnia.

Red Light Therapy – Bring the healing power of natural light into your nighttime routine. Red light therapy mimics the wavelengths of a natural sunset, signaling the body to wind down and produce melatonin. This NASA-backed technology has been shown to improve sleep efficiency, reduce sleep latency, and regulate the circadian rhythm, making it a revolutionary tool for deep, restorative sleep.

Sleep science is evolving, and so should you. These revolutionary recovery technologies are reshaping how we rest, repair, and rejuvenate. Whether you're looking to train your brain, supercharge cellular healing, or regulate your circadian rhythm, these cutting-edge tools offer new pathways to deeper, higher-quality sleep and optimal well-being.

Jane's Journey to Restful Nights

For years, Jane had battled a relentless enemy – insomnia. At sixty-five, she found herself trapped in an exhausting cycle: staring at the ceiling for hours, waking up groggy, and feeling drained before the day even began. No matter how tired she was, her mind refused to shut down, racing with endless thoughts. Night after night, she longed for the deep, restorative sleep that had once come so easily.

Jane didn't buy the idea that poor sleep was just part of getting older. Determined to reclaim her nights, she committed to a structured bedtime routine, incorporating gentle relaxation techniques, mindful breathing, and the soothing power of sleep-inducing rituals. She swapped late-night screen time for a warm cup of chamomile tea, replaced stress with guided meditation, and trained her body to associate bedtime with peace, not frustration.

Then, something surprising happened! For the first time in years, Jane drifted into effortless, restorative sleep – no tossing, no turning, just deep, uninterrupted rest. Her mornings transformed: she woke up feeling refreshed, her energy levels soared, and her mind felt sharper and clearer than ever. The fog of exhaustion lifted, and with it, she rediscovered the joy of waking up with purpose and vitality. Even in later life, quality sleep is within your reach. Jane's story is proof that with the right approach – a structured routine, relaxation techniques, and a commitment to sleep hygiene – it's possible to overcome insomnia and unlock the rejuvenating power of deep sleep.

Mark's Experience with Sleep Technology: Unlocking Restorative Sleep at Seventy-Two

At seventy-two, Mark was a relentless entrepreneur, a visionary who had spent decades building businesses, chasing innovation, and pushing his limits. But despite his success, there was one battle he couldn't seem to win – his sleep.

For years, his nights were restless, filled with fragmented sleep cycles that left him feeling drained, foggy, and
unfocused during the day. Late-night work sessions, constant mental stimulation, and the stresses of entrepreneurship had taken a toll. He had convinced himself that "sleep
is for the weak," but deep down, he knew his productivity
and longevity depended on solving this problem.

Then, Mark turned to technology. He started wearing a
high-tech sleep tracker, a device that analyzed his sleep
patterns in real time. The results were eye-opening: his
deep sleep was severely lacking, and his body wasn't getting the restorative rest it desperately needed.

Determined to make a change, Mark implemented
these small but strategic adjustments: He reduced late-
night work, shutting down screens an hour before bed to
allow his brain to unwind. He introduced a white noise
machine, blocking out disruptive sounds and creating a
sleep-inducing environment. He embraced a structured
nighttime routine, signaling to his body that it was time to
rest.

The results? Transformational. Within weeks, Mark's
deep sleep increased by 40 percent; his mornings felt clearer, more energized, and more productive than ever before.
His mental sharpness returned, his stress levels dropped,
and for the first time in years, he felt like he had reclaimed
control over his well-being. Technology isn't just for tracking steps – it can unlock the secrets of better sleep. By analyzing sleep data and making small, intentional changes,
Mark proved that even at seventy-two, it's possible to optimize sleep, boost recovery, and enhance cognitive function for a longer, healthier life.

Robert's Weighted Blanket Success: From Rest-
less Nights to Deep, Restorative Sleep

For years, Robert's nights were anything but restful.
The moment he lay down, his mind refused to quiet – endless thoughts, worries, and anxieties swirled in his head like

an unstoppable storm. No matter how exhausted he felt, sleep remained elusive.

He tried everything – meditation, herbal teas, cutting back on caffeine – but nothing seemed to work. Tossing and turning became his nightly routine, frustration mounting as the hours slipped away. Each morning, he woke up feeling drained, unfocused, and trapped in a cycle of exhaustion.

Then, he discovered the power of deep pressure stimulation – a concept that would transform his sleep. Skeptical yet desperate for a solution, Robert decided to try a weighted blanket. He wasn't sure what to expect, but as soon as he pulled it over him, something surprising happened. The gentle, even pressure wrapped around him like a cocoon, easing the tension in his body almost instantly. His breathing slowed, his muscles relaxed, and for the first time in years, he felt a sense of deep calm. That night, he fell asleep faster than he ever had before. The weighted blanket worked like a natural sleep aid, lowering stress hormones, increasing serotonin, and signaling to his body that it was safe to rest. Night after night, his sleep became deeper, longer, and more restorative.

What was once a struggle had become a sanctuary. The weighted blanket wasn't just a sleep accessory – it was a life-changing tool that gave Robert back the peace he had been searching for. Anxiety-induced restlessness doesn't have to define your nights. With the help of a weighted blanket, deep, uninterrupted sleep is within reach – bringing comfort, security, and the restorative power of true relaxation.

Final Thoughts: Sleep – The Ultimate Key to a Longer, Healthier Life If you have ever assumed that poor sleep is just part of getting older, it's time to think again. Sleep is a foundational pillar of longevity, vitality, and overall well-being. Far beyond simple rest, it's a dynamic biological process that repairs tissues, balances hormones, clears toxins from the brain, and restores every cell in your body.

Far more than just rest, sleep is an active, biological process that rejuvenates every cell in your body. While you sleep, your brain undergoes a powerful detoxification process, flushing out harmful toxins linked to neurodegenerative diseases like Alzheimer's. Your DNA is actively repaired, preserving the integrity of your genetic blueprint. Hormones that regulate metabolism, immune function, and stress are balanced, ensuring your body operates at its peak.

On the other hand, sleep deprivation is a silent accelerator of aging. It disrupts cognitive function, weakens the immune system, and increases the risk of chronic illnesses such as heart disease, diabetes, and dementia. Every hour of missed sleep chips away at longevity, robbing you of the energy, clarity, and resilience that define a long and fulfilling life.

The good news? Optimizing your sleep is one of the easiest, most powerful longevity strategies available. With the right habits – a structured sleep routine, a supportive environment, and mindful light exposure – you can unlock deeper, more restorative sleep that fuels your body's ability to heal, grow, and thrive. Your longevity journey starts tonight – with a great night's sleep. Prioritize rest, embrace its power, and watch as it transforms not only your nights but the quality and length of your life.

CHAPTER 7:
STRESS MANAGEMENT
AND MENTAL RESILIENCE

"A calm mind is the ultimate tool for a long and fulfilled life."
— Maria L. Ellis, BBA, MBA

Emely never expected to feel old in her fifties. Emily had always been the woman in control – commanding boardrooms by day and hosting dinner parties by night – but something started to shift. First, it was the brain fog – small things, like forgetting passwords or zoning out during high-level meetings. Then came the fatigue. Not the kind a good night's sleep could fix, but a deep, dragging weariness that clung to her even on weekends. Her face looked different in the mirror too – tired, puffy, somehow older.

At first, she chalked it up to age. But deep down, she knew this was more than aging – it was accelerated aging, and something was driving it.

That something was chronic stress. Emily had been living in a state of near-constant pressure for years – endless deadlines, late-night emails, nonstop decision-making. Her body had adapted by producing more cortisol, the stress hormone that helps in short bursts but becomes damaging when it's always elevated. What Emily didn't know then was that cortisol, when left unchecked, does more than just keep you up at night – it quietly wreaks havoc on your body at the cellular level.

Chronic stress shrinks the hippocampus, the brain's memory center, and impairs cognitive function. It raises inflammation, which contributes to everything from heart disease to wrinkles. It disrupts insulin sensitivity, making it harder to maintain a healthy weight. And it interferes with sleep, robbing the body of its natural repair cycle. Over time, all of this adds up – not just to burnout, but to biological aging far beyond your actual years.

Emily began to see it. She wasn't just tired – she was running on fumes. Her hair was thinning. Her digestion was off. Her skin had lost its glow. She was aging from the inside out, and stress was the accelerator. But that realization was her turning point.

Emily's turning point came one afternoon in the middle of a meeting she would've normally led with ease. Her thoughts kept slipping. She couldn't find the words she needed, and for the first time in her career, she panicked in front of her team. That night, she cried in the car before driving home. Not because of one bad day, but because she realized how long she'd been running on empty.

That was the night she said to herself, "This is not who I want to be. This is not how I want to live." So Emily did something radical – for her, at least. She took a week off. No laptop. No phone. Just quiet time to breathe, reflect, and reset. At first, it felt uncomfortable. Her nervous system was so wired she didn't know how to rest. But slowly, things began to shift.

She started practicing deep breathing – just five minutes in the morning, eyes closed, hands on her heart. It wasn't dramatic, but it helped. Her body stopped bracing. Her mind softened. She started journaling in the evenings, letting the racing thoughts out onto paper instead of letting them swirl in her head. She began protecting her sleep like it was a sacred appointment, creating a calm nighttime ritual with herbal tea, soft music, and no screens after nine p.m.

And most importantly, she learned to say no. She created boundaries around her time, her availability, and her energy. She stopped overcommitting. She gave herself permission to rest – not as a reward, but a right.

The result? Within three months, Emily was sleeping better, smiling more, and showing up to work with clarity and confidence again. Her doctor noticed improvements in her blood pressure and inflammation markers. Even her friends said she looked more radiant – like she'd come back to life.

Emily's story is powerful because it reminds us that you don't need a total life overhaul to slow the aging process – you just need intentional moments of pause, protection, and presence. Chronic stress can be sneaky. It can disguise itself as ambition or responsibility. But your body always knows – and it will speak in symptoms long before you consciously register the need to slow down. You don't have to wait for a breakdown to begin your breakthrough.

The Hidden Impact of Stress on Aging

Stress is often considered an unavoidable part of life – a natural response to challenges, uncertainty, and change. In small doses, stress can be beneficial, sharpening our focus and preparing us to take action. But when stress becomes chronic, it shifts from being a helpful ally to a silent but powerful force that accelerates aging, damages our health, and diminishes our quality of life.

Many people associate longevity with exercise, nutrition, and sleep, but few realize that managing stress is just as critical to living a long, healthy life. Chronic stress is a biological disruptor, affecting every system in the body – from the brain and heart to the immune system and even our DNA.

When we experience prolonged stress, our body continuously releases cortisol, a hormone meant to help us respond to immediate threats. However, elevated cortisol over time contributes to inflammation, oxidative stress, and the shortening of telomeres – the protective caps on our DNA that determine lifespan. Scientists have even found that stress can alter brain structure, increasing the risk of cognitive decline and neurodegenerative diseases.

The good news is that stress is not just something that happens to us; it is something we can learn to manage. Developing mental resilience – the ability to adapt, stay calm under pressure, and recover quickly from setbacks – can help slow the aging process, improve overall well-being, and even extend our lifespan.

This chapter explores the profound impact of stress on aging and longevity, revealing the scientific mechanisms at play and providing practical, evidence-based strategies to build resilience. By mastering the art of stress management, we can protect our health, sharpen our minds, and create a life filled with greater peace, purpose, and longevity. Let's explore how we can take control of stress before it takes control of us.

How Chronic Stress Accelerates Aging

Stress, in small doses, can be beneficial – it prepares our bodies for "fight or flight" situations and can enhance focus. However, when stress becomes chronic, it turns from a survival mechanism into a silent killer. When the body is under stress, it releases cortisol, a hormone that is vital for acute stress responses. However, prolonged cortisol exposure can lead to a host of problems, including increased blood pressure, insulin resistance, and impaired immune function. Elevated cortisol levels also interfere with the production of growth hormone – a key player in tissue repair and regeneration – which accelerates the aging process.

Chronic stress fuels ongoing, low-grade inflammation. Inflammatory cytokines released during stress damage cells, contribute to the formation of plaques in arteries, and can disrupt the normal functioning of various organs.

Over time, this inflammation accelerates the wear and tear on our bodies, leading to conditions like cardiovascular disease, arthritis, and even neurodegenerative disorders. Chronic stress disrupts the balance between free radicals and antioxidants, making it harder for the body to repair itself. Free radicals can damage DNA, proteins, and lipids, resulting in premature cell aging. This oxidative stress is a key factor in the development of age-related diseases and contributes to the shortening of telomeres – the protective caps on our chromosomes that naturally shorten with age. Telomeres protect our genetic material during cell division. Studies have shown that individuals exposed to prolonged psychological stress exhibit significantly shorter telomeres, indicating that stress accelerates the aging process on a cellular level. Shortened telomeres have been linked to a host of age-related conditions, including heart disease, diabetes, and certain cancers.

The Brain on Stress: Cognitive Decline and Emotional Turbulence

The brain is particularly sensitive to stress. The constant bombardment of stress hormones not only impacts memory and learning but also changes the very structure of the brain. The hippocampus, a critical region for memory and learning, is one of the first areas to be affected by chronic stress. High cortisol levels can lead to the shrinkage of this region, resulting in memory impairment and difficulty in forming new memories. This deterioration is a key factor in age-related cognitive decline and increases the risk of dementia.

The amygdala is the brain's center for processing emotions such as fear and anxiety. Under chronic stress, the amygdala becomes overactive, heightening emotional responses and making it harder to regulate mood. This persistent state of anxiety not only undermines mental wellbeing but also perpetuates a cycle of stress that further accelerates aging. The prefrontal cortex is responsible for executive functions such as decision-making, attention, and self-control. Chronic stress can impair how this region functions, reducing one's ability to think clearly and make sound decisions. Over time, this cognitive impairment can lead to decreased productivity, poor judgment, and an overall decline in quality of life.

The immune system is another victim of chronic stress. When the body is constantly in a state of alert, the immune response is compromised. Stress-induced cortisol release suppresses the immune system, reducing the production of antibodies and increasing vulnerability to infections. Chronic stress leads to an overproduction of inflammatory markers, which not only impair immune function but also contribute to the progression of chronic diseases.

Cultivating Mental Resilience: Tools for Stress Management

Given the profound impact of stress on both our bodies and minds, developing strategies to manage stress is essential. Building mental resilience – the ability to adapt and recover – is a lifelong practice that can dramatically improve your quality of life and longevity. Mindfulness is the practice of staying present and fully engaged with the current moment without judgment. Meditation, as a structured form of mindfulness, has been shown to reduce stress and promote mental clarity.

Scientific Evidence Behind Mindfulness

Numerous studies have shown that regular meditation practice lowers cortisol levels, thereby mitigating the harmful effects of chronic stress. Mindfulness meditation has been linked to increased thickness in the prefrontal cortex and reduced activity in the amygdala, promoting emotional regulation and improved cognitive function. Emerging research suggests that mindfulness practices may help maintain telomere length, providing a cellular shield against aging. Incorporating daily mindfulness practices such as meditation for ten to twenty minutes using guided apps like Headspace or Calm, mindful breathing exercises to regulate stress, and body scans to release tension and promote relaxation can significantly enhance mental clarity, emotional balance, and overall well-being.

Cognitive Behavioral Techniques

Cognitive Behavioral Therapy (CBT) is a well-established method for changing negative thought patterns that contribute to stress. While traditionally used in clinical settings, the core principles of CBT can be applied in everyday life to build resilience. The first step is to become aware of the automatic negative thoughts that arise in response to stress. Write them down if needed.

Challenging Cognitive Distortions:

Question the validity of these thoughts. Are they based on facts or assumptions? Replace them with more balanced, rational perspectives. Engage in activities that counteract stress. This might include hobbies, exercise, or socializing – anything that brings joy and a sense of accomplishment. Trying journaling to spot stress patterns, reframing setbacks as growth moments, and listing three things you're grateful for each day can significantly improve emotional resilience, reduce stress, and cultivate a more positive and balanced mindset.

Physical Activity as a Stress Reliever

Exercise is one of the most powerful and natural stress relievers, as it triggers endorphin release to elevate mood, improves sleep quality to enhance recovery, and boosts cognitive function by increasing blood flow to the brain, all of which help reduce anxiety, enhance mental clarity, and provide a healthy outlet for stress management. Incorporating practical exercise strategies such as aerobic activities like walking or cycling for at least thirty minutes a day to reduce stress, strength training to build both physical and mental resilience, and mindful practices like yoga and Tai Chi to enhance overall balance and relaxation can significantly improve emotional well-being and promote long-term health.

Social Connections and Community Support

Humans are inherently social beings, and strong social connections serve as a powerful buffer against stress by fostering emotional support, stimulating oxytocin release to build trust and reduce anxiety, enabling cognitive reframing to gain new perspectives on challenges, and preventing isolation, which is a key contributor to accelerated aging and mental distress.

Rest and Recovery Practices

Rest isn't just about sleep – it's about incorporating periods of recovery into your daily routine to allow your mind and body to rejuvenate. Prioritizing downtime is essential for stress management and overall well-being, whether through active recovery activities like reading or spending time in nature, digital detoxes to give the mind a break from constant stimulation, or structured relaxation techniques such as progressive muscle relaxation and guided imagery to lower tension and promote inner calm. Incorporating practical relaxation strategies such as scheduled breaks throughout the day to step away from stress, engaging in mindful leisure activities like gardening or painting to restore energy, and establishing an evening wind-down routine with reading, stretching, or a warm bath can significantly enhance mental clarity, reduce stress, and improve overall well-being.

Developing a Personal Stress-Management Plan

Every individual is unique, and so is the way they experience and manage stress. Creating a personalized plan that integrates multiple strategies can lead to lasting change and improved resilience. Consider the following steps when designing your own plan:

Developing self-awareness is the foundation of effective stress management, starting with identifying your stressors – whether they stem from work, relationships, or finances – by journaling to recognize patterns and monitoring how your body and mind react, such as experiencing headaches or muscle tension, to gain a deeper understanding of your personal stress response.

Establishing healthy routines is key to long-term stress management, including daily mindfulness or meditation to lower baseline stress levels, regular physical activity that combines aerobic, strength, and flexibility exercises, and a balanced diet rich in antioxidants and omega-3s to nourish the body and support brain health – ensuring resilience against daily stressors.

Building a Support Network

Building a strong support network is essential for managing stress. That might mean nurturing uplifting social connections or working with a therapist who can offer personalized guidance through life's challenges.

Embracing Rest and Recovery

Embracing rest and recovery is essential for overall well-being, which includes prioritizing quality sleep by maintaining a consistent schedule and creating a restful environment, as well as planning regular downtime for leisure activities, hobbies, and relaxation to restore both body and mind. Effective stress management requires regular check-ins with yourself – noticing changes in mood, energy, and well-being, and adjusting your approach as life shifts.

Real-Life Stories of Transformation

To truly understand the power of stress management and mental resilience, consider these real-life examples:

Case Study: Emily's Journey to a Calmer Mind

At fifty-eight years old, Emily was at the peak of her career as a high-level executive in a fast-paced corporate environment. Her days were a whirlwind of back-to-back meetings, endless emails, and mounting responsibilities, leaving her with little time to breathe – let alone focus on self-care. The relentless pressure took a toll on her well-being, manifesting in sleepless nights, chronic anxiety, and a sharp decline in both her physical and mental health.

Despite her professional success, Emily felt like she was constantly running on empty. She experienced frequent headaches, muscle tension, and digestive issues – clear signs that stress was taking a toll on her body.

Her once-sharp focus began to fade, replaced by a persistent brain fog that made even simple decisions feel overwhelming. She knew something had to change.

One evening, while attending a corporate wellness seminar, she heard about the scientifically proven benefits of mindfulness meditation. Though initially skeptical – how could sitting in silence possibly help her manage the chaos? – she decided to give it a try.

Emily started small, setting aside just fifteen minutes each morning for a guided meditation session using a mindfulness app. At first, her mind raced uncontrollably, and she struggled to sit still. But as the days passed, she noticed subtle yet profound shifts: her breathing slowed, her thoughts became clearer, and she approached her workday with a newfound sense of control and calm.

Within weeks, the changes became undeniable. Her sleep improved, allowing her to wake up refreshed and energized rather than drained. Her cortisol levels decreased, reducing the chronic inflammation that had plagued her for years. The constant tightness in her shoulders eased, and her ability to navigate stressful situations with composure transformed both her professional and personal life.

As mindfulness became a cornerstone of her daily routine, Emily found herself making other positive changes as well – she began prioritizing short breaks throughout the day, practicing deep breathing before high-stakes meetings, and even inspiring her colleagues to explore stress-management techniques.

Looking back, Emily marvels at how such a simple practice created such a profound transformation. What once felt like an unstoppable cycle of stress and burnout had been replaced with balance, clarity, and resilience. Emily's story is a powerful testament to the fact that small, intentional changes – like dedicating a few minutes to mindfulness each day – can have life-changing effects on stress levels, mental clarity, and overall well-being.

Case Study: Robert's Transformation Through Cognitive Restructuring

At sixty-five years old, Robert should have been enjoying the golden years of retirement, yet he found himself trapped in a cycle of negativity and anxiety. Having spent decades in a demanding corporate career, he had always tied his self-worth to his productivity, and now, without a structured work routine, he felt lost, restless, and uncertain about his future.

The creeping thoughts of aging, lost opportunities, and an uncertain purpose weighed heavily on him. Every minor inconvenience felt like proof that life was slipping away, and he often caught himself dwelling on past mistakes or worrying excessively about the future. The anxiety affected his relationships, making him withdrawn and irritable, and his sleep suffered as his mind raced through endless worst-case scenarios.

Recognizing that his mental patterns were holding him back, Robert decided to seek help. He began working with a therapist trained in cognitive-behavioral therapy (CBT), a method designed to help individuals recognize and reframe irrational thoughts. Initially, he resisted the idea that changing his thinking could change his reality – after all, wasn't aging just a slow decline?

But as he committed to the process, something incredible happened. Through structured exercises, Robert learned to identify negative thought loops and challenge them with logic and evidence. Instead of thinking, "I'm too old to try something new," he began replacing it with, "I have decades of wisdom and experience that can help me explore new opportunities." When he caught himself believing, "I'm a burden to my family," he consciously reframed it to "My presence, support, and stories enrich my loved ones' lives."

The transformation was nothing short of remarkable.

With each passing week, his mindset shifted from one of fear to one of possibility. He began saying yes to social invitations, rekindling old friendships and exploring new ones. His relationships flourished, as he was no longer weighed down by self-doubt and negativity. His sleep improved, his energy levels increased, and most importantly, he felt a renewed sense of purpose.

Looking back, Robert was struck by how much of his suffering had come from his thoughts – not the reality around him.

Robert's journey proves that our thoughts shape our reality. By actively challenging and reframing negative beliefs, he reclaimed control over his emotional well-being, strengthened his relationships, and found new meaning and purpose in his later years – a true testament to the power of cognitive restructuring in promoting longevity and happiness.

Case Study: Sandra's Path to Resilience Through Social Connection

At seventy years old, Sandra found herself facing a loneliness she had never known before. After losing her husband of forty-five years, the once vibrant home they had built together felt empty and unbearably silent. Grief weighed heavily on her, and isolation only deepened her sadness. Her daily routines, once shared with her spouse, now felt meaningless, and she often spent days without speaking to anyone.

As weeks turned into months, her emotional distress began affecting her physical health – she experienced fatigue, trouble sleeping, and a persistent sense of sadness. Even simple tasks, like making meals or going for a walk, felt overwhelming. She knew something had to change – but she didn't yet know how to rebuild after such a profound loss.

One afternoon, while visiting the local library, she saw a flyer for a community group for seniors that met weekly for social activities, book discussions, and shared hobbies. The thought of walking into a room full of strangers terrified her, but something deep inside urged her to give it a try.

The first meeting was nerve-wracking, but as she listened to others share their stories – some of whom had also experienced loss – she felt a sense of belonging she hadn't felt in months. Slowly, she started to open up, sharing pieces of her own journey, and in doing so, she realized that she was not alone. With each passing week, Sandra grew stronger. She joined a book club, where lively discussions reignited her love for literature and intellectual engagement. She discovered a passion for gardening, finding peace and purpose in nurturing life once more. She attended community events, laughing more than she had in years, and forming deep, meaningful friendships with others who truly understood her journey.

The loneliness that had once consumed her began to fade, replaced by genuine connections, a renewed sense of purpose, and the comforting knowledge that she was part of a community that cared. Her stress levels declined, her energy returned, and she slept more soundly, no longer burdened by the heavy weight of isolation. One evening, after a particularly joyful book club discussion, she reflected on how far she had come. She realized that healing hadn't come from simply "moving on" but from moving forward – with people who supported and uplifted her.

Sandra's journey is a testament to the healing power of social connection. By taking a courageous step to re-engage with her community, she not only managed her stress and overcame loneliness but also found joy, resilience, and a new purpose in life – proving that no one is ever truly alone when they seek the company of kindred spirits.

Integrating Stress Management into Daily Life

To show how mastering stress and recovery can truly transform a life, let me share a chapter from my own journey. During my years as a corporate lending officer, I was traveling for business development, managing a portfolio of demanding corporate accounts, and raising two children at the same time. Life moved at a relentless pace – early morning flights, late-night client meetings, endless deadlines, and the constant pull of family responsibilities. I was driven and successful, but beneath the surface, I was running on adrenaline and slowly burning out. It wasn't until I discovered simple but powerful techniques – like pausing for a few minutes of breathwork before high-stakes meetings, using mindfulness to center myself between appointments, and deliberately carving out moments for active recovery – that my health began to shift. These small daily practices helped me manage my stress, reclaim my energy, and protect my well-being without sacrificing my ambitions or my family life. Looking back, I realize these strategies were not just survival tactics – they were the foundation for sustainable success and longevity.

Integrating stress management into daily life starts with small, intentional rituals. Try meditative breathing to center the mind, gratitude journaling to build positivity, and light stretching or yoga to awaken the body – helping to build resilience and set a balanced tone for the day ahead.

Incorporating mindful breaks throughout the day –

such as taking a five-minute walk to refresh the mind, using a quick meditation app to ease tension, or practicing deep breathing exercises to lower stress levels – helps prevent burnout, enhance focus, and maintain a sense of calm amidst daily responsibilities.

Ending your day with intentional wind-down practices – such as a digital detox to reduce screen exposure, reflective journaling to process thoughts and appreciate daily wins, or engaging in relaxing hobbies like reading, listening to gentle music, or taking a warm bath – helps calm the mind, ease stress, and promote restorative sleep for better overall well-being.

Final Thoughts: A Calm Mind for a Longer, Richer Life

While stress is an inevitable part of life, the way we manage it shapes our health, happiness, and longevity. By adopting a holistic approach – prioritizing mindfulness and meditation to lower cortisol, engaging in cognitive behavioral strategies to foster resilience, staying physically active to enhance well-being, nurturing social connections for emotional support, and integrating rest and recovery to restore balance – we empower ourselves to live not just longer, but with greater vitality, peace, and fulfillment.

Ultimately, a calm mind is more than a state of tranquility – it is the foundation upon which a long, vibrant, and resilient life is built. By making stress management and mental resilience central to your daily routine, you are not only protecting your health but also enriching every moment of your life.

Take these lessons to heart. Every moment you spend nurturing your mental well-being is an investment in your longevity. As you progress on this journey, know that each small step brings you closer to a more peaceful, balanced, and fulfilling existence.

This chapter is designed to be both informative and practical, offering a comprehensive look at the science behind stress and longevity while equipping you with actionable strategies to cultivate a calm, resilient mind. Embrace these practices, and let your journey to a long, healthy life begin with the power of a peaceful mind.

In closing this chapter, let's Reflect + Take Action: Reclaiming Calm, One Step at a Time. Reflection Questions:

Have you noticed signs of stress in your body – like fatigue, brain fog, tension, or trouble sleeping? What are they trying to tell you?

Are there responsibilities or pressures you've taken on that no longer serve your health or happiness?

When was the last time you felt truly rested, both mentally and physically? What would it take to experience that more often?

Emily's Stress Recovery Checklist – Try One Today! A Five-Minute Breathwork: Start your day with five slow, deep breaths in and out, with your hand over your heart. Screen-Free Wind-Down: Turn off electronics one hour before bed and create a soothing nighttime ritual. Journal Your Mind: Spend a few minutes at night writing down thoughts that are cluttering your mind. Say "No" Gently: Choose one small thing to decline this week, and use that time to rest or recharge. Move to Release: Go for a ten-minute walk, dance to music you love, or stretch to release tension from your body.

Chronic stress may be invisible, but its impact on your body and your aging process is very real. The good news is, just like Emily, you have the power to slow that process – and even reverse it – by choosing rest, setting boundaries, and inviting stillness into your life. This isn't about weakness. It's about wisdom. It's about listening to your body before it starts shouting. You deserve to feel calm, clear, and in control again. And with each small shift you make, you're not just protecting your health – you're reclaiming your joy. Let's keep going. Your next breakthrough is just ahead.

CHAPTER 8:
THE IMPACT OF SOCIAL CONNECTIONS ON LIFESPAN

*"No man is an island entire of itself; every man
is a piece of the continent, a part of the main.".*

— John Donne

It was after her husband passed that Lorraine started to fade. Not physically at first – her health was steady – but emotionally. Her days felt quieter, her meals lonelier, and her laughter far less frequent. Her doctor noted no immediate red flags, but something was missing. "I just don't feel like myself anymore," she said one day, eyes cast down. "I go through the motions, but I'm not really living."

Then something small changed everything. Her daughter signed her up for a weekly art class at the local community center. Lorraine didn't want to go at first, but she went. She met others. She painted. She laughed. After a few weeks, her energy lifted. She started walking to class instead of driving. She began cooking again – real meals, not just toast. Her blood pressure improved, her sleep deepened, and most importantly, she felt connected again.

Lorraine didn't find her spark in a supplement or a health trend – she found it in connection: shared stories, gentle encouragement, and laughter. And that's where we turn next, because longevity isn't just about what you eat or how you move – it's also about who you surround yourself with.

The Power of Connection for a Long, Healthy Life

In the pursuit of longevity, we often focus on diet, exercise, and medical advancements. Yet one of the most powerful and overlooked factors in extending lifespan is human connection. Our relationships – whether with family, friends, or our broader community – shape not only our emotional well-being but also our physical health and resilience against disease.

For centuries, philosophers and scientists alike have emphasized the importance of social bonds. John Donne's famous words, "No man is an island," ring true now more than ever. Modern research confirms what many cultures have long understood: those with strong social ties live longer, healthier, and more fulfilling lives.

But what happens when social connections are lacking? Loneliness and isolation have been linked to increased mortality rates, cognitive decline, and chronic diseases. In fact, studies show that prolonged loneliness is as harmful to health as smoking fifteen cigarettes a day. In contrast, individuals who maintain strong social relationships experience lower stress levels, improved immune function, and a reduced risk of age-related illnesses like Alzheimer's and heart disease.

Though we often credit longevity to diet and exercise, human connection may be the most powerful – and most overlooked – factor of all. The quality of our relationships has a profound effect on our mental, emotional, and physical health.

People with strong social bonds live longer, healthier, and more fulfilling lives. Studies show that meaningful relationships help lower stress levels, strengthen the immune system, reduce the risk of cognitive decline, and increase overall well-being.

Conversely, loneliness and social isolation are as detrimental to health as smoking fifteen cigarettes a day, leading to increased risks of heart disease, depression, and even premature death.

In this chapter, we'll explore the science behind connection and longevity – how relationships shape our health, the dangers of isolation, and practical ways to build meaningful bonds.

The goal is to not just live longer, but to live with joy, purpose, and companionship. Let's dive into how relationships shape our longevity.

A Tale of Two Lives: The Power of Relationships in Action

To illustrate the impact of relationships on longevity, the study closely followed two participants:

William: The Isolated Intellectual

William, a brilliant lawyer, excelled in his career but prioritized work over relationships. He gradually lost touch with friends and family, becoming increasingly isolated in his fifties. By his late sixties, he reported chronic stress, poor sleep, and declining cognitive function. Despite being financially successful, he suffered from early heart disease and depression, and by his seventies, he struggled with severe health issues.

John: The Socially Engaged Optimist

John, on the other hand, wasn't a top student or a wealthy businessman, but he nurtured lifelong friendships and maintained close family ties. He regularly engaged in community activities, had deep, meaningful conversations with loved ones, and leaned on his social network for emotional support during tough times. At eighty, John remained mentally sharp, physically active, and content with life, with a lower incidence of disease compared to his peers.

Though John faced challenges too, his strong relationships helped him manage stress, stay resilient, and age more gracefully. Meanwhile, William's lack of meaningful social bonds accelerated his decline.

The Science Behind Relationships and Longevity

Human connection isn't just beneficial – it's a biological necessity. Social interactions influence a wide range of physiological processes, from reducing inflammation to enhancing brain function.

The Longevity Benefits of Social Interaction

Reduces Stress and Lowers Cortisol Levels

Chronic stress contributes to high blood pressure, inflammation, and an increased risk of heart disease. Strong relationships trigger the release of oxytocin – the bonding hormone that naturally lowers stress. This helps lower cortisol levels, reducing the harmful effects of chronic stress.

A study published in Psychosomatic Medicine found that people with strong social ties had lower blood pressure and heart rates, suggesting that close relationships serve as a buffer against stress-related diseases.

Boosts Immune Function and Speeds Up Recovery

People with strong relationships tend to have stronger immune systems, recover faster from illnesses, and have a lower risk of infections.

In a study published in Health Psychology, researchers found that people with more social support produced higher levels of antibodies in response to vaccines, meaning their immune systems were more robust.

Improves Cognitive Health and Reduces Risk of Dementia

Social engagement keeps the brain active and stimulated, reducing the risk of cognitive decline. A Harvard Medical School study found that seniors who engaged in regular conversations and social activities had a 70 percent lower risk of developing Alzheimer's disease compared to those who were socially isolated.

Dr. Benjamin Carter, a neuroscientist at Harvard Medical School, had dedicated his career to studying the human brain and the mysteries of aging. For years, he had examined the biological markers of Alzheimer's disease, searching for patterns that could explain why some seniors remained sharp well into their eighties and nineties, while others experienced rapid cognitive decline.

His latest research led him to a groundbreaking discovery – one that confirmed what many had long suspected but had never been fully quantified: seniors who regularly engaged in conversations and social activities had a 70 percent lower risk of developing Alzheimer's compared to those who were socially isolated.

Dr. Carter's study followed thousands of elderly participants over two decades, meticulously tracking their lifestyle habits, cognitive function, and social interactions. The findings were unmistakable – those who maintained active social lives, whether through friendships, family interactions, community involvement, or even casual conversations with neighbors, showed remarkable resilience against cognitive decline.

Behind the data were real people – older adults who protected their minds not with medication, but with meaningful connection.

Encouraging Healthy Habits and Accountability: The Power of Social Influence on Longevity

We are social creatures by nature, and the people we surround ourselves with significantly impact our daily habits, lifestyle choices, and overall health. Research has shown that social circles influence everything from diet and exercise to sleep patterns and even our willingness to seek medical care.

When we engage with health-conscious individuals, we are far more likely to exercise regularly and stay active, eat nutritious foods and make better dietary choices, engage in preventive health care and screenings, and maintain a positive mindset and manage stress effectively. In contrast, individuals who are socially isolated or surrounded by unhealthy influences are more likely to adopt poor habits, experience higher stress levels, and neglect their health.

But why is this the case? Let's dive into the science behind social influence and accountability in health and how we can use it to our advantage for a longer, healthier life.

The Science Behind Social Influence on Healthy Habits

Research shows that our habits are contagious – for better or worse – as we tend to mirror the behaviors of those around us. This concept, known as behavioral contagion, means that we subconsciously adopt the habits and attitudes of the people around us.

The Framingham Heart Study, a landmark study on social networks and health, found that if a friend becomes obese, your chances of becoming obese increase by 57 percent. If a friend quits smoking, your likelihood of quitting rises significantly. If a close contact engages in regular physical activity, you are more likely to exercise. The people in our social circles influence our decisions more than we realize. If we surround ourselves with individuals who prioritize health, we naturally adopt healthier behaviors as well.

The Role of Accountability: Why We Stay on Track When Others Are Watching

Accountability plays a huge role in sticking to long-term health goals. When we commit to a goal publicly or with a group, we are far more likely to follow through.

Imagine these two scenarios:

Scenario 1: Walking Alone

You set a personal goal to walk 10,000 steps a day.

Some days, you feel motivated, but on others, you skip the walk, telling yourself, "I'll make up for it tomorrow." Over time, your motivation fades, and the habit disappears.

Scenario 2: Walking with a Friend or Group

You and a friend commit to a morning walk every day at seven a.m. Even when you don't feel like going, you don't want to let your friend down. The expectation of meeting someone keeps you accountable, and the habit sticks.

Studies show that people who engage in group activities or have accountability partners are significantly more likely to achieve their health goals. This applies to diet, exercise, sleep, stress management, and even regular medical checkups.

How Social Circles Influence Diet and Nutrition

The Social Effect of Eating Habits

Have you ever gone out to eat with a group of friends and noticed that your food choices are influenced by what others order? If your friends order fast food, you're more likely to do the same. If they opt for healthy meals, you're more inclined to follow suit. A study published in Appetite found that people tend to match the eating habits of those they dine with, often consuming more vegetables and making healthier choices when surrounded by health-conscious peers.

Real-World Example: The Blue Zones

In Okinawa, Japan, one of the world's longest-living communities, people form lifelong social groups called "moai." These groups meet regularly to eat meals together, exercise, and support one another emotionally.

As a result, Okinawans maintain healthy eating habits for life, contributing to their low rates of heart disease, obesity, and dementia. When we share meals with people who prioritize nutrition, we naturally adopt healthier eating habits.

You can apply this in your own life by hosting healthy potlucks where friends bring nutritious, home-cooked meals; planning social outings around wellness, like going for a walk or meeting for a smoothie instead of drinks; and surrounding yourself with people who value nutrition, so their healthy habits naturally influence your own.

Staying Physically Active with Supportive Friends

One of the biggest barriers to consistent exercise is lack of motivation. However, when we engage in physical activity with others, we are much more likely to stay committed. A study published in the Journal of Social Sciences found that people who exercise with friends or in groups are 60 percent more likely to maintain an active lifestyle. Working out with a more advanced partner improves performance and motivation. Fitness levels of close friends tend to be similar – active friends encourage each other to keep moving.

Some of the benefits of group workouts include more motivation – exercising with friends makes workouts more enjoyable and sustainable; accountability – knowing someone expects you makes you more likely to show up; better performance – friendly competition pushes you to challenge yourself; and social bonding – builds friendships while improving health.

You too can apply this to your life by joining a fitness class – yoga, dance, Pilates, or cycling classes foster social bonds; finding a workout partner – a walking, jogging, or gym buddy can help keep you accountable; participating in local health groups – join a walking group, hiking club, or recreational sports league. Surrounding yourself with active individuals increases your likelihood of staying active, too.

Encouraging Preventive Health and Medical Check-ups

People who are socially connected are more likely to seek medical care, engage in preventive screenings, and follow doctors' recommendations. A study from the

American Journal of Public Health found that people with strong social support are 30 percent more likely to attend annual check-ups and screenings. Women with close friends are more likely to get mammograms and other preventive tests. Men with supportive social networks are more likely to monitor their blood pressure and cholesterol levels.

Encouragement and reminders from loved ones play a crucial role. If your spouse, friend, or family member nudges you to schedule a check-up, you're more likely to do it. You can apply this to your life by reminding loved ones to schedule check-ups, encourage health screenings and preventive care, and hold each other accountable for following medical advice. Social support makes us more proactive about our health, reducing the risk of undiagnosed illnesses.

The Power of Positive Influence

The people we surround ourselves with shape our behaviors, choices, and ultimately, our longevity. By engaging with health-conscious, active, and supportive individuals, we increase our chances of living a longer, healthier life.

Some of the key takeaways include habits that mirror those of your closest friends and family. Being part of a health-conscious community leads to better lifestyle choices.

Accountability partners keep you motivated and on track. Preventive care is more likely when social circles emphasize health. Choose your circle wisely – your relationships are one of the most powerful determinants of your health and lifespan. Longevity is not just about genetics – it's about relationships. Surrounding yourself with supportive people can literally add years to your life.

The Science of Longevity and Social Connections

Scientists have identified four key mechanisms through which relationships influence longevity: Stress Reduction – Lower cortisol levels decrease inflammation and improve cardiovascular health; Healthier Behaviors – Friends and family help encourage positive lifestyle habits; Stronger Immune System – Social connections enhance immune function, reducing disease risk; and increased Sense of Purpose – A sense of belonging and purpose is linked to lower mortality rates.

The Harvard Study of Adult Development: The Strongest Predictor of Longevity and Happiness

One of the most remarkable and longest-running studies on human health and well-being is the Harvard Study of Adult Development. Spanning over eighty years, this study has provided some of the most compelling evidence that close relationships – not wealth, fame, or genetics – are the strongest predictor of long-term health and happiness.

In the 1930s, Harvard researchers began tracking the lives of 268 male Harvard undergraduates, later expanding the study to include inner-city residents and their descendants, ultimately following over 2,000 individuals across multiple generations. Researchers regularly collected data on their physical health, mental well-being, career paths, relationships, and personal struggles.

The key finding? The quality of social connections was the most significant factor in predicting health, longevity, and life satisfaction – even more than income, social class, IQ, or lifestyle habits. The Harvard Study of Adult Development found that close, high-quality relationships are the strongest predictor of long-term health, happiness, and longevity, as they reduce chronic disease, lower stress and inflammation, protect brain function, lessen physical pain, and increase overall life satisfaction, whereas social isolation accelerates cognitive decline, raises the risk of heart disease and depression, and diminishes emotional well-being.

Why Do Relationships Have Such a Powerful Effect on Health?

The Harvard study, along with other research, has identified several biological and psychological reasons why relationships are essential for longevity.

Relationships Reduce Stress and Lower Cortisol Levels

Chronic stress drives inflammation, strains the heart, and accelerates cognitive decline. Supportive relationships act as a buffer against stress, helping to regulate cortisol levels. When people feel emotionally secure, their bodies remain in a state of balance rather than prolonged fight-or-flight mode. Studies show that hugging a loved one or having a deep conversation reduces cortisol levels and increases oxytocin, a hormone that promotes relaxation and trust.

Social Connections Strengthen the Immune System

Lonely individuals experience higher levels of inflammation, which weakens the immune system and increases the risk of disease. In contrast, people who are socially active produce more antibodies and recover from illness faster. A study from Carnegie Mellon University found that people with strong social networks were less likely to catch the common cold, even when exposed to the virus.

Good Relationships Promote Heart Health

Strong marriages, close friendships, and supportive family ties are all linked to lower rates of heart disease. Emotional support helps regulate blood pressure, cholesterol levels, and heart rate variability, reducing the risk of strokes and heart attacks. Research from the American Heart Association found that individuals in happy marriages had a 50 percent lower risk of cardiovascular disease.

Social Engagement Keeps the Brain Active

Conversations, shared activities, and emotional bonding help maintain neural connections in the brain, reducing the risk of Alzheimer's and dementia. Socially isolated individuals experience faster cognitive decline and brain shrinkage. Studies show that engaging in frequent social interactions increases the production of brain-derived neurotrophic factor (BDNF), a protein essential for brain health and memory retention.

A Sense of Purpose Extends Life

People with strong social ties often feel a greater sense of meaning and purpose, which has been linked to lower mortality rates and improved overall well-being. Having responsibilities – whether as a friend, spouse, mentor, or community member – gives people a reason to stay mentally and physically active. Blue Zones – regions known for exceptional longevity – reveal that socially connected individuals live, on average, eight to ten years longer than their isolated peers.

How to Apply the Harvard Study's Findings to Your Own Life

The Harvard Study of Adult Development provides a clear blueprint for longevity: Prioritize Relationships Over Work and Material Success – Invest time in family, friends, and deep conversations rather than chasing superficial achievements. Nurture a Small Circle of Meaningful Connections – Quality matters more than quantity. Having a few deep, supportive relationships is more beneficial than hundreds of shallow ones. Engage in Social Activities and Join Communities – Participate in book clubs, fitness groups, or local meetups to build social bonds. Check In Regularly with Loved Ones – Small gestures like phone calls, weekly dinners, or handwritten notes strengthen relationships. Develop Intergenerational Friendships – Learning from elders and mentoring younger people fosters purpose and keeps the mind sharp. Be a Support System for Others – Acts of kindness not only improve someone else's life but also boost your well-being.

Final Thoughts: Relationships Are the Greatest Predictor of a Long, Fulfilling Life

The Harvard Study of Adult Development confirms the truth that we often overlook: that a good life is built on good relationships. It turns out it's not wealth, status, or even intelligence that determines how long – or how well – we live. It's not just about diet or exercise; it's about who we share our lives with. Meaningful relationships lower stress, protect the brain, and keep us physically healthy.

So as you plan for longevity, ask yourself: Who do I spend the most time with? Am I nurturing my relationships? How can I create more social connections? The quality of your relationships today will determine the quality of your health and happiness decades from now. Prioritize connection, and you'll not only live longer – you'll live better.

This eighty-year study, one of the longest-running in history, found that close relationships were the strongest predictor of long-term health and happiness – even more than genetics or lifestyle habits.

Case Study: The Alameda County Study – The Longevity Power of Social Connections

In the quest for longevity, diet and exercise often get the spotlight – but one of the strongest predictors of a long, healthy life may actually be the strength of your relationships.

A groundbreaking nine-year study in Alameda County, California, tracked thousands of participants to uncover the impact of social connections on longevity. The findings were nothing short of remarkable: individuals with strong social ties had significantly lower mortality rates, living longer, healthier lives than those who were socially isolated. Social isolation was as detrimental to health as smoking, obesity, and lack of exercise, increasing the risk of chronic disease, cognitive decline, and premature death. Those who engaged in regular social interactions – whether through family, friends, or community activities – showed lower levels of stress, stronger immune function, and greater emotional resilience.

The Science Behind Social Longevity

Human connection is more than just emotional fulfillment – it has measurable physiological benefits. Heart Health: Socially connected individuals have lower blood pressure, reduced inflammation, and a lower risk of cardiovascular disease. Cognitive Protection: Meaningful relationships stimulate the brain, lowering the risk of dementia and Alzheimer's disease. Stronger Immunity: A rich social life boosts immune function, reducing susceptibility to illness and chronic disease. Lower Stress and Anxiety: Engaging with loved ones reduces cortisol (the stress hormone) and increases feel-good neurotransmitters like oxytocin and serotonin. Connection is Longevity Medicine.

The Alameda County Study proves that a strong social network is just as essential for health and longevity as proper nutrition and exercise. Prioritizing relationships, engaging in community, and nurturing deep connections isn't just good for the soul – it's a scientifically backed strategy for living a longer, healthier, and more vibrant life. Longevity isn't just about how you eat or move – it's about who you share your life with. Investing in meaningful relationships is one of the most powerful ways to extend your lifespan, protect your health, and ensure a fulfilling, joyful existence.

The Roseto Effect: How Community Protects the Heart and Extends Life

In the rolling hills of Pennsylvania, a small town held a medical mystery that defied conventional wisdom. In the mid-twentieth century, researchers turned their attention to Roseto, a close-knit Italian-American community where residents were living longer, healthier lives – despite indulging in high-fat, high-cholesterol diets, smoking, and consuming wine regularly.

What they discovered was astonishing: Roseto had remarkably low rates of heart disease, strokes, and stress-related illnesses. Compared to neighboring towns, where cardiovascular disease was a leading cause of death, Rosetans were practically immune. The secret? It wasn't their diet – it was their way of life.

The Science Behind the Roseto Effect

Rather than nutrition or genetics, researchers found that Roseto's heart-protective power came from its deeply rooted sense of community. Strong Social Bonds: Families in Roseto lived together across multiple generations, offering constant emotional and financial support. Frequent Social Gatherings: Residents regularly ate meals together, attended church, and participated in community celebrations, reducing loneliness and stress. Low Social Competition and High Belonging: Unlike in many modern societies, in Roseto, success wasn't measured in wealth or status, but in relationships, rituals, and mutual support. They supported one another, shared resources, and valued relationships over material gain. Lower Stress Levels: The town's emphasis on social cohesion and emotional support resulted in lower blood pressure, reduced cortisol levels, and stronger immune function. Community is Heart Medicine.

The Roseto Effect proves that meaningful human connections are just as essential to longevity as diet and exercise. In a world where stress, isolation, and social disconnection are on the rise, Roseto serves as a powerful reminder that strong relationships, emotional support, and a sense of belonging are protective factors against disease. The heart thrives on connection. The Roseto Effect shows us that nurturing relationships, fostering a sense of belonging, and embracing a supportive community are powerful, science-backed longevity strategies that can add years to our lives – and life to our years.

The Dangers of Social Isolation

Loneliness is a silent killer, increasing the risk of early death, cognitive decline, and emotional distress. Loneliness isn't just painful – it increases early death risk by 50%, weakens immunity, and doubles the likelihood of Alzheimer's.

Practical Ways to Strengthen Community and Relationships

Building strong social connections doesn't have to be complicated. Here are simple, practical ways to cultivate meaningful relationships. Building strong social connections is simple yet powerful – prioritizing family and close friendships through regular meetups, expressing gratitude, and engaging in shared activities like exercise, travel, or cooking can strengthen bonds, enhance well-being, and create a lasting sense of belonging.

Joining Social Groups and Longevity Communities

Joining social groups and longevity communities by volunteering, participating in wellness or hobby groups, and building intergenerational friendships fosters a sense of purpose, emotional resilience, and lifelong engagement, all of which contribute to a longer, healthier, and more fulfilling life.

Real-Life Stories of Longevity Through Relationships

John's Journey: Finding Purpose Through Volunteering

For thirty-five years, John had thrived in the fast-paced world of corporate finance. His days were filled with meetings, problem-solving, and mentoring young professionals. But when he retired at sixty-seven, the once-exhilarating structure of his life vanished overnight.

At first, he enjoyed the freedom – no alarm clocks, no deadlines – but soon, a deep sense of emptiness crept in. The purpose that had fueled his daily routine was gone, and loneliness became his unexpected companion. Days blurred into weeks, and he found himself sitting at home, watching television, reminiscing about the past, and struggling to find fulfillment in this new phase of life.

One day, while attending a community event, John struck up a conversation with a young entrepreneur struggling to navigate the complexities of business ownership. As they talked, John felt something ignite within him – his knowledge and experience, which he had thought were relics of the past, suddenly had real value.

Encouraged by this encounter, John joined a local mentorship program, offering guidance to aspiring entrepreneurs. At first, he committed to just a few hours a week, but he soon found himself immersed in the energy, ambition, and fresh perspectives of the younger generation. His days regained structure, his mind stayed sharp, and most importantly, he felt needed again.

Over time, John built lasting friendships with many of the young entrepreneurs he mentored. They not only benefited from his wisdom, but they also introduced him to new ideas, technologies, and even social activities he had never considered. He attended networking events, joined business forums, and found himself once again surrounded by passionate, driven individuals – just as he had in his working years.

His happiness and energy levels soared. He felt reconnected to the world, proving that retirement doesn't have to mean slowing down – it can be a doorway to new opportunities, relationships, and purpose.

John's story demonstrates that purpose is a crucial component of longevity. By staying engaged in meaningful work, building new social connections, and sharing his knowledge, he not only extended his life but enriched it as well.

Sarah's Social Circle: How a Walking Group Changed Her Life

At seventy years old, Sarah found herself in a completely new environment – a city where she knew no one, surrounded by unfamiliar streets and empty days. Having recently relocated to be closer to her daughter and grandchildren, she had expected to feel a sense of belonging and excitement. Instead, loneliness set in.

She missed the comfort of familiar faces, the daily chats with neighbors, and the simple routines that had shaped her life for decades. Her once-active social life had vanished, replaced by quiet afternoons spent alone. The isolation weighed on her, affecting both her mood and motivation.

One afternoon, while browsing the community center's bulletin board, she spotted a flyer:

"Sunrise Strollers: A Walking Group for Seniors – Meet New Friends, Stay Active, and Enjoy the Outdoors!"

Something about it intrigued her. She hadn't been very active in recent years, but the idea of fresh air and friendly company was appealing. With hesitation and a bit of nervous excitement, she decided to attend her first walk the next morning.

When she arrived, a warm, welcoming group of seniors greeted her. Some had been part of the group for years, others were newcomers just like her. As they set off on the tree-lined walking trail, conversation flowed effortlessly. They talked about everything – from books and travel to their families and favorite recipes.

What began as a simple daily walk became a lifeline. Sarah quickly found herself bonding with her fellow walkers – sharing laughter, swapping stories, and offering support during life's ups and downs. The group became her extended family, filling the void she had felt since moving.

Physically, she noticed incredible changes. The daily walks improved her energy levels, strength, and even her sleep. Her once-aching joints felt more limber, and she moved with newfound confidence.

Emotionally, the transformation was even greater. Gone were the lonely afternoons. She now had weekly lunch outings, group excursions, and a circle of friends who genuinely cared for one another.

One day, while enjoying coffee after a walk, Sarah reflected on how different she felt compared to just a few months earlier. She had come to the city seeking family, and she found one – not just in her daughter's home, but within a group of kindred spirits who walked beside her, quite literally, every step of the way.

Sarah's story reminds us that even one small step toward connection can transform our health, happiness, and sense of belonging. By taking one small step – joining a walking group – she transformed her health, happiness, and sense of belonging, proving that it's never too late to build meaningful relationships and embrace a new chapter in life.

Miguel and Maria: The Power of Lifelong Love

Miguel and Maria's love story began over five decades ago, in a small coastal town where they first met as young dreamers with big ambitions and even bigger hearts. From the moment they exchanged glances at a local festival, their connection was effortless, filled with warmth, laughter, and an unspoken understanding.

Now, at seventy-five and seventy-three, they look back on their journey together, knowing that love and companionship have been the greatest gifts to their health and longevity. While many wonder about the secret to a long, happy life, Miguel and Maria firmly believe that it lies in the strength of their relationship – not just in their commitment to one another, but in their shared experiences, daily habits, and unwavering support.

The Science of Love and Longevity

Studies show that married couples or those in strong, loving relationships live longer, experience lower levels of stress, and have better heart health. The Harvard Study of Adult Development even found that good relationships keep us healthier and happier more than money, career success, or genetics. Miguel and Maria are living proof of this reality.

Prioritizing Communication and Emotional Support

From the start, Miguel and Maria understood that communication was the foundation of their love. They made a pact early in their marriage: never go to bed angry. Even during disagreements, they would sit together, talk it out, and find common ground.

"We may not always agree," Maria says with a smile, "but we always listen to each other. And that has made all the difference."

This open and honest communication has helped them navigate life's ups and downs – raising children, facing financial struggles, adjusting to retirement – without letting stress consume them. The result? A calmer mind, a healthier heart, and a stronger connection.

Engaging in Shared Activities for Physical and Mental Well-Being

Unlike some couples who gradually drift into separate routines over time, Miguel and Maria have always prioritized togetherness, whether it's taking morning walks along the beach to start their day with fresh air and conversation, practicing gentle yoga for flexibility and mental clarity, cooking Mediterranean-inspired dishes that nourish both body and soul, challenging each other with brain games to stay sharp, or dancing in their living room to keep their youthful spirit alive – proving that shared activities not only strengthen their bond but also contribute to their longevity and happiness.

The Healing Power of Laughter and Playfulness

If there's one thing that sets Miguel and Maria apart, it's their ability to find joy in the simplest moments. Miguel is a storyteller, often filling their evenings with humorous tales from their younger days, while Maria has a quick wit that keeps their conversations lively and full of laughter. They tease each other playfully, turning even mundane moments – like folding laundry – into a shared joke. Their laughter is infectious, uplifting, and, most importantly, healing. Science confirms that laughter lowers stress hormones, boosts immune function, and releases endorphins, the body's natural mood boosters. "Our secret?" Miguel chuckles. "Never take life – or each other – too seriously."

Weathering Life's Storms Together

Of course, life hasn't always been easy. There were hardships, losses, and moments of doubt, but through it all, they remained each other's anchor.

When Miguel faced health issues in his sixties, Maria became his fiercest advocate, ensuring he received the best care while keeping his spirits high. When Maria struggled with the transition into retirement, Miguel encouraged her to find new passions, explore hobbies, and embrace the change as a new adventure.

Their ability to adapt, support, and grow together has given them a resilience that few couples achieve.

The Results: A Life Well-Lived, Together

Now, after fifty years of marriage, Miguel and Maria wake up each morning grateful for another day by each other's side. Their strong relationship has lowered their stress levels, kept them physically active and engaged, protected their heart and brain health, and provided them with a lifelong source of joy and purpose. "Love doesn't just make life more beautiful," Maria says. "It makes it longer, healthier, and worth every single moment."

Miguel and Maria's story proves that love isn't just about romance – it's about deep connection, shared laughter, mutual support, and growing together. Their commitment to each other is a testament to the power of companionship in longevity, showing us that a life filled with love is not just a longer life – it's a richer, more fulfilling one.

The Key to a Longer, More Fulfilling Life

The research is clear: human connection is a fundamental pillar of longevity, as strong relationships reduce stress, strengthen immunity, and encourage healthier behaviors, while loneliness poses a serious health risk, increasing disease and mortality – proving that prioritizing social connections not only adds years to life but also fills those years with joy, purpose, and well-being. In summary, your diet, exercise routine, and sleep habits matter – but so do your relationships. Invest in your social health just as you would in your physical health, and you'll create a life that is not just long but deeply fulfilling. This chapter makes social connection a priority in longevity, providing science-backed evidence and real-world strategies.

CHAPTER 9:
THE FUTURE OF ANTI-AGING THERAPIES AND BREAKTHROUGH TREATMENTS

"Tomorrow's longevity solutions begin with today's innovations."
— Maria L. Ellis, BBA, MBA

The world of anti-aging science is advancing faster than ever, with promising breakthroughs emerging in areas like senolytic drugs, stem cell therapies, gene editing, and cellular rejuvenation. These treatments aim not just to extend lifespan, but to increase health span – the years we live with mobility, clarity, and vitality.

Take senolytic therapy, for example. These treatments target and remove senescent cells – cells that have stopped functioning but linger in the body, promoting inflammation and aging. In a recent clinical trial, patients over seventy who received a short course of senolytics experienced measurable improvements in muscle strength and stamina. One participant, Jane, seventy-five, shared that for the first time in years, she was able to return to her gardening hobby without feeling drained the next day. "It was like my body finally had a little more life in it," she said.

Another area gaining momentum is NAD+ restoration therapy, aimed at replenishing a coenzyme critical to energy production and DNA repair. While this therapy is still being refined, early adopters – especially those over sixty – report enhanced mental clarity and fewer midday energy crashes. David, sixty-eight, a retired engineer, noticed that after several weeks of NAD+ supplementation, he no longer needed his afternoon nap and was back to writing code for fun – something he hadn't done in years.

Gene therapies, once the stuff of science fiction, are now entering early clinical trials. In one such study, researchers introduced a gene modification that enhanced mitochondrial function in aging mice – restoring youthful strength and endurance. The implications for humans are still under exploration, but the potential is real and deeply hopeful.

These stories remind us that we're on the cusp of a new era. Yes, many of these treatments are still in development – but the trajectory is clear. What once felt like science fiction is becoming the foundation of next-generation healthcare. And what that means for you is simple, yet profound: aging well is no longer just about managing decline – it's about proactively restoring what time has taken.

The Next Frontier in Longevity

What if aging was no longer inevitable? What if science could slow, halt, or even reverse the aging process at its very core? These are no longer science fiction fantasies – they are real possibilities on the horizon of longevity science.

The field of anti-aging and regenerative medicine is advancing at an unprecedented pace. Leading scientists, visionary researchers, and biohackers around the world are racing to unlock the secrets of cellular rejuvenation, genetic optimization, and age-reversing interventions. These breakthroughs are redefining human health, offering the potential to extend lifespan, enhance vitality, and push the boundaries of what it means to age.

From gene-editing technologies like CRISPR to senolytics that clear out aging cells, and from stem cell therapies to AI-driven diagnostics that predict disease before it manifests, the future of aging is being rewritten in real-time. The possibilities are extraordinary – and they're already beginning to change lives.

This chapter will take you on a journey into the future of longevity, exploring the most promising anti-aging therapies and the real-life stories of those who are already benefiting from these groundbreaking innovations. The next era of human health is not just about living longer – it's about living better, stronger, and more vibrantly than ever before. Welcome to the future of aging, where science meets possibility, and longevity is no longer a dream but a reality in the making.

The Most Promising Anti-Aging Therapies

Senolytics: Clearing Out Zombie Cells Senolytics are therapies that eliminate senescent or 'zombie' cells – dysfunctional cells that accumulate with age and drive inflammation and disease. Senolytics are a class of therapies designed to target and eliminate senescent cells, also known as "zombie cells." These cells accumulate as we age and contribute to inflammation, disease, and overall physical decline. Unlike normal cells, senescent cells refuse to die, lingering in the body and releasing toxic chemicals that damage surrounding healthy cells. Research has shown that removing these cells can enhance physical function, extend lifespan, and reduce age-related diseases. Here are a few powerful examples of how senolytic therapy is already changing lives. Senolytic drugs selectively remove aged cells, reducing inflammation and improving tissue function. Studies show that removing senescent cells can extend lifespan and improve mobility in animal models.

Case Study 1: Richard's Return to Strength

At seventy-eight, Richard had accepted that his body was slowing down. Once an avid hiker, he now found it difficult to climb even a single flight of stairs without experiencing joint pain and breathlessness. His doctor informed him that his body was accumulating senescent cells, contributing to his chronic inflammation and fatigue.

After enrolling in a clinical trial for senolytic therapy, Richard began a regimen that targeted and eliminated these "zombie cells." Within three months, he felt a significant difference. His mobility improved, inflammation decreased, and he found himself able to walk longer distances without pain. For the first time in years, he set a goal to return to hiking – and within six months, he was back on the trails.

Case Study 2: Margaret's Mental Clarity

Margaret, seventy-four, had always prided herself on her sharp mind. But over the years, she noticed she was forgetting names, losing track of conversations, and struggling with mental fog. Her energy levels had dropped, and she felt sluggish even after a full night's sleep.

After reading about the connection between senescent cells and cognitive decline, she decided to try a natural senolytic supplement containing quercetin and fisetin, compounds known for their ability to clear out aging cells. Within weeks, Margaret noticed a shift: clearer thinking, sharper focus, and more sustained energy. She was no longer struggling to keep up in conversations and felt a renewed sense of confidence in her memory.

Case Study 3: David's Recovery from Joint Pain

David, eighty-one, had suffered from debilitating arthritis for years. His knees were swollen, and even standing for long periods left him in agony. Conventional pain treatments only provided temporary relief, and he worried that he would soon be unable to move without assistance.

His physician recommended a combination of senolytic drugs and lifestyle changes to target the buildup of senescent cells in his joints. Within a few months, David's inflammation significantly decreased, and he regained his ability to move freely. For the first time in years, he no longer needed painkillers to get through the day.

What This Means for Longevity

These stories highlight the remarkable potential of senolytics in reversing some of the most debilitating effects of aging. By actively removing toxic, aging cells from the body, senolytics open the door to a future where people can live healthier, longer, and more active lives. As research continues, more therapies and supplements are emerging, offering hope for those suffering from chronic pain, cognitive decline, and age-related diseases. The key to longevity isn't just extending life – it's ensuring those extra years are filled with vitality and well-being. Could senolytics be the missing piece in the puzzle of aging? For many, the answer appears to be yes!

Gene Therapy: Reprogramming the Aging Process

Gene therapy aims to modify or repair damaged DNA to slow aging and prevent age-related diseases.

Case Study 1: Michael's Reversal of Muscle Degeneration

Michael, a sixty-nine-year-old retired engineer, had always been active, but over the past decade, he noticed a significant loss of muscle strength. Simple activities like lifting groceries or getting up from a chair had become challenging. His doctor diagnosed him with sarcopenia, an age-related muscle deterioration, and warned that it would only get worse.

Desperate for a solution, Michael enrolled in a gene therapy trial that targeted the MYOSTATIN gene, a gene responsible for regulating muscle growth. By selectively inhibiting this gene, the therapy reignited his body's natural ability to build muscle. Within six months, Michael saw a dramatic improvement – his muscles regained strength, his endurance increased, and for the first time in years, he could jog without pain. The results were profound: Michael rebuilt muscle strength, regained endurance, and significantly lowered his risk of falls and fractures.

Case Study 2: Evelyn's Fight Against Cognitive Decline

At seventy-five, Evelyn had started experiencing memory lapses. Forgetting names, misplacing items, and struggling to recall important dates became daily frustrations. Her family noticed the changes and feared the early signs of dementia.

Evelyn's doctor introduced her to gene therapy targeting the APOE4 gene, a key genetic marker linked to Alzheimer's disease. The therapy worked by modifying the expression of protective genes that enhanced her brain's ability to clear harmful plaques and regenerate neurons. Within eight months, Evelyn's cognitive function had significantly improved. She was more alert, more engaged in conversations, and no longer feared losing herself to dementia. This gene therapy helped Evelyn to improve memory retention and focus,

reduce the buildup of harmful brain plaques, and increase neuronal regeneration and cognitive longevity.

Case Study 3: James' Regeneration of Joint Cartilage

For years, James, eighty, struggled with severe osteoarthritis. The pain in his knees made walking excruciating, and doctors suggested knee replacement surgery. Instead, James opted to try gene therapy designed to regenerate cartilage tissue.

Using CRISPR-based gene editing, scientists activated his COL2A1 gene, which plays a key role in producing cartilage. Over the next few months, James noticed an incredible transformation – his joint pain disappeared, mobility returned, and inflammation subsided. He was able to walk pain-free for the first time in over a decade.

The Future of Gene Therapy in Longevity

Gene therapy has moved from science fiction to reality, offering promising solutions to combat aging at the genetic level. As research continues, scientists are developing therapies to extend telomeres, protect DNA from deterioration, enhance mitochondrial function, increase energy and metabolism, and regrow damaged organs, providing a new frontier in regenerative medicine. The ability to reprogram the body's aging process is no longer a dream – it's happening now. As more breakthroughs emerge, gene therapy has the potential to not only extend lifespan but also enhance the quality of life for millions around the world.

CRISPR and Genetic Editing – Scientists are exploring ways to repair damaged genes linked to aging.

Case Study 1: Jennifer's Battle Against Premature Aging

Jennifer, a fifty-year-old woman, had always looked older than her age due to a rare genetic condition that caused rapid telomere shortening. Doctors informed her that her cells were aging at nearly twice the normal rate, leading to brittle bones, chronic fatigue, and early onset arthritis. Through a cutting-edge CRISPR gene-editing therapy, scientists were able to restore her telomerase activity, essentially reversing the premature shortening of her telomeres. Over the next year, Jennifer experienced increased energy, stronger bones, and improved skin elasticity. More remarkably, her biological age markers suggested she had gained back nearly a decade of youth at the cellular level.

Case Study 2: Robert's Recovery from Genetic Heart Disease

At sixty-two, Robert had already suffered one mild heart attack due to a genetic mutation in the PCSK9 gene, which led to dangerously high cholesterol levels. Despite leading a healthy lifestyle, he was at high risk for another, more severe cardiac event. After enrolling in a CRISPR gene-editing clinical trial, Robert's defective PCSK9 gene

was permanently silenced, reducing his LDL (bad cholesterol) levels by more than 50 percent within three months.
His doctor informed him that he now had the cardiovascular profile of someone twenty years younger. Robert was
able to lower his cholesterol without lifelong medication,
reduce his heart attack risk by modifying genetic predisposition, and improve his cardiovascular health without major lifestyle changes.

***Case Study 3: Maria's Fight Against Neurodegen-
eration***

Maria, a retired professor, had a strong family history
of Alzheimer's disease. At sixty-seven, she began noticing
subtle memory lapses and difficulty concentrating, which
worried her deeply. Genetic testing confirmed she carried
two copies of the APOE4 gene, increasing her risk of developing Alzheimer's by over twelve times the normal rate.
Through an experimental CRISPR-based gene therapy,
doctors modified her APOE4 gene to behave more like
APOE2, a protective variant found in people resistant to
Alzheimer's. Over the following year, Maria's cognitive
decline slowed significantly, and new brain scans showed a
reduction in amyloid plaque buildup.

She not only regained her mental sharpness but felt
empowered by taking proactive control of her cognitive
future.

The Future of CRISPR and Genetic Editing in Longevity

These case studies highlight the transformative potential of CRISPR and genetic editing to repair damaged
genes, prevent disease, and slow the aging process. Scientists are now exploring gene therapy applications that
could extend lifespan by targeting aging-related genes, regenerating damaged tissues and organs, and reversing age-
related decline at the cellular level. As gene-editing technology advances, the future of longevity is shifting from
simply managing symptoms to curing aging at its genetic

root. The potential to edit out genetic diseases, optimize cellular function, and reprogram human aging itself is no longer science fiction – it's becoming a reality.

Gene Therapy for Longevity

Early studies suggest it could potentially extend human lifespan by targeting aging-related genes.

Stem Cell Therapy: Regenerating Tissues and Organs

Stem cell therapy is one of the most exciting areas of anti-aging research. By replacing old or damaged cells with fresh stem cells, the body can repair tissues, regenerate organs, and even reverse some effects of aging. Stem cells show promise in treating arthritis, neurodegenerative diseases, and even skin rejuvenation – all while enhancing immune function and slowing age-related decline.

Case Study 1: John's Journey to Joint Regeneration

At seventy-four, John had resigned himself to a life of limited mobility. His severe osteoarthritis had worn away the cartilage in his knees, making every step painful. Doctors recommended joint replacement surgery, but John was reluctant to undergo such an invasive procedure.

Desperate for an alternative, he explored stem cell therapy, which involved injecting mesenchymal stem cells (MSCs) into his knees to promote cartilage regeneration. Within months, he noticed a remarkable improvement: his pain diminished, and his mobility steadily returned.

Case Study 2: Emily's Heart Repair

Emily, a sixty-eight-year-old retired nurse, suffered a heart attack that left her with severe damage to her cardiac tissue. Traditional medicine could only offer symptom management, but Emily wanted to heal.

She enrolled in a stem cell therapy trial that used cardiac stem cells to regenerate damaged heart tissue. Over the following months, scans revealed that her heart function was improving, her energy levels were rising, and she no longer experienced the constant fatigue that had plagued her since the heart attack.

Case Study 3: Mark's Recovery from Spinal Cord Injury

At fifty-five, Mark was left partially paralyzed after a car accident damaged his spinal cord. Doctors told him he might never regain full movement, but Mark refused to accept that prognosis.

He participated in a stem cell trial where neural stem cells were implanted into his spinal cord to regenerate damaged nerves. Slowly, feeling returned to his legs. After a year of therapy and rehabilitation, he could stand and take assisted steps – a feat once deemed impossible.

The Future of Stem Cell Therapy

Stem cell research is revolutionizing the way we approach aging and disease. Scientists are exploring how stem cells can regenerate organs, heal injuries, and reverse degenerative conditions. The future may hold even greater advancements, including regenerating liver tissue to reverse liver disease, rebuilding pancreatic cells to treat diabetes, and repairing damaged brain tissue in stroke survivors.

Breakthroughs in stem cell therapy are bringing longer, healthier lives within reach. These real-life success stories prove that regenerative medicine is not just about adding years to life – but restoring the ability to truly live.

NAD+ Therapy: Boosting Cellular Energy and Rewiring Aging at the Molecular Level

Aging, at its core, is a battle against cellular decline – a slow deterioration of mitochondrial function, metabolic efficiency, and DNA integrity. But what if we could replenish the fuel that powers our cells, restoring vitality, enhancing endurance, and extending health span? This is where NAD+ (Nicotinamide Adenine Dinucleotide) therapy steps in as one of the most promising breakthroughs in longevity science.

As a biohacker, I incorporate NAD+ supplementation into my regimen, experiencing firsthand its impact on energy metabolism, mitochondrial performance, and overall vitality. The results have been nothing short of transformative. By boosting NAD+ levels through precursors like NMN (Nicotinamide Mononucleotide) or NR (Nicotinamide Riboside), I've noticed enhanced cellular energy – no more mid-day crashes or persistent fatigue. Sharper mental clarity – improved focus, memory, and cognitive endurance. Faster recovery – my body feels stronger, more resilient, and quicker to recover from stress.

The Science Behind NAD+ and Longevity

NAD+ is a coenzyme found in every cell, playing a vital role in energy production, DNA repair, and cellular defense mechanisms. However, as we age, NAD+ levels drop drastically, leading to slower metabolism, mitochondrial dysfunction (cellular fatigue), accumulated DNA damage (faster aging at a cellular level), and increased susceptibility to age-related diseases.

By supplementing with NAD+ precursors, we can reignite cellular function, enhancing mitochondrial health, reducing fatigue, and supporting longevity at the molecular level.

Real-Life Case Studies: The Transformative Power of NAD+ Therapy

Athletes and biohackers: Professional athletes and performance-driven individuals are using NAD+ to accelerate recovery, boost endurance, and optimize metabolic efficiency.

Longevity researchers and scientists: Visionary scientists in the field of aging, like Dr. David Sinclair, have touted NAD+ as a key player in reversing cellular aging and extending health span. Everyday people seeking vitality: Individuals in their forties, fifties, and beyond are incorporating NAD+ to restore youthful energy, fight cognitive decline, and maintain metabolic health well into old age. With ongoing research exploring NAD+ infusions, optimized precursor formulations, and its role in disease prevention, the future of harnessing this powerful molecule for longevity is just beginning. NAD+ therapy represents a powerful tool for restoring cellular energy and resilience. By replenishing this critical coenzyme, we can slow the aging process, optimize mitochondrial health, and sustain youthful energy for decades to come.

Case Study 1: Sarah's Return to Vitality

At sixty-seven, Sarah felt constantly drained, no matter how much sleep she got. She had always been an active person, but in recent years, she found herself struggling with low energy, brain fog, and muscle weakness. Her doctors chalked it up to aging, but she knew there had to be more to it. After learning about NAD+ therapy, Sarah decided to try it. NAD+ (Nicotinamide Adenine Dinucleotide) is a coenzyme essential for cellular energy production, and levels naturally decline with age. Within weeks of receiving NAD+ IV infusions, Sarah noticed remarkable improvements – her energy levels increased, her cognitive function sharpened, and she felt decades younger.

Case Study 2: David's Recovery from Chronic Fatigue

For years, David, seventy-two, had battled chronic fatigue syndrome, making even simple tasks feel exhausting. His doctors had tried everything, from dietary changes to medications, but nothing seemed to work. When a longevity specialist suggested NAD+ therapy, he was skeptical but willing to try. David began a protocol of NAD+ supplementation combined with lifestyle modifications, including better sleep hygiene and intermittent fasting. Within months, his energy levels surged. He no longer needed afternoon naps, could exercise without feeling depleted, and even resumed his passion for woodworking.

Case Study 3: Linda's Fight Against Cognitive Decline

At seventy-four, Linda started experiencing mild memory loss and difficulty concentrating. While her doctor assured her this was normal aging, she was determined to take control of her cognitive health. She discovered research linking NAD+ therapy to brain function and decided to try it. Through NAD+ IV treatments and supplementation, Linda saw significant cognitive improvements. Her memory sharpened, her ability to focus increased, and she felt more engaged in conversations. Follow-up scans confirmed increased neuronal activity, supporting the role of NAD+ in slowing cognitive decline.

The Future of NAD+ Therapy

As research advances, NAD+ therapy is becoming a cornerstone of longevity science. Scientists are exploring its potential in enhancing metabolic health and reversing insulin resistance, improving muscle recovery, reducing inflammation, lowering age-related DNA damage, and extending lifespan. By restoring NAD+ levels, individuals are not just increasing their lifespan – they are improving their quality of life, ensuring they have the energy, clarity, and vitality to enjoy the years ahead.

AI-Powered Longevity and Personalized Medicine

Artificial intelligence is revolutionizing preventative healthcare and longevity medicine by analyzing genetic data, lifestyle factors, and biomarkers to create personalized anti-aging strategies.

Case Study 1: James' AI-Optimized Health Transformation

At sixty-five, James had been struggling with unexplained fatigue, high cholesterol, and irregular sleep patterns. Despite following a conventional health plan, he saw little improvement. Frustrated, he turned to an AI-powered longevity platform that used real-time biomarker tracking and predictive analytics to optimize his health. Using wearable technology and AI-driven insights, James received a personalized nutrition and exercise plan tailored to his genetic makeup. Within six months, he experienced increased energy, improved metabolic health, and deeper sleep. His cholesterol levels dropped naturally without medication, and his biological age (measured by epigenetic testing) reversed by five years.

Case Study 2: Sophia's AI-Guided Cancer Prevention

At fifty-eight, Sophia had a family history of breast cancer and wanted to take proactive steps to reduce her risk. Instead of waiting for symptoms, she used an AI-driven early detection platform that analyzed her genetic markers, lifestyle, and hormone fluctuations to create a custom risk profile. The AI system flagged early warning signs of cellular abnormalities long before conventional screenings would have detected them. With this insight, Sophia worked with a longevity specialist to modify her diet, supplement intake, and hormone balance. Two years later, follow-up tests showed her cellular health had significantly improved, and her cancer risk had dropped by 40 percent.

Case Study 3: David's AI-Personalized Drug Therapy

David, seventy-two, had been diagnosed with Parkinson's disease, and despite traditional treatments, his symptoms continued to progress. Frustrated with trial-and-error medications, he enrolled in an AI-powered personalized medicine program. Using machine learning algorithms, the system analyzed David's genetic profile, lifestyle habits, and response to previous medications to create a customized treatment plan. The AI model adjusted his medication dosages, recommended alternative supplements, and optimized his daily schedule for peak energy and brain function. Within months, David's tremors decreased, his speech improved, and he regained mobility. His doctors were astonished at how well his body responded when treatment was precisely aligned with his genetic needs.

The Future of AI in Longevity

AI is revolutionizing personalized medicine, preventative care, and longevity science. As technology advances, "AI-powered tools will predict disease before symptoms arise, optimize drug regimens using real-time data, and customize lifestyle plans to maximize both lifespan and health span." AI-driven longevity medicine is not just extending life – it's ensuring those extra years are lived in optimal health, energy, and vitality.

As a biohacker, I also take STEMREGEN, a natural advanced stem cell support to boost my body's natural ability to repair and regenerate itself. Cellular Repair Therapy: NanoVi® Oxidative Stress Relief helps prevent and reverse cellular damage by supporting protein folding and cellular resilience. Glutathione Therapy: Supplementation with Auro Wellness Glutathione supports detoxification, enhances immune resilience, and promotes healthy cellular aging. T.A. Sciences TA-65 Supplement helps activate telomerase, promoting healthy cellular function and slowing the aging process.

Final Thoughts: A New Era in Aging

We are entering an age where living to be older than 100 and in good health is becoming a real possibility. These breakthrough therapies offer hope, innovation, and the potential to dramatically improve quality of life as we age. While these treatments are still evolving, they represent a glimpse into a future where aging is not something to fear but something to manage and optimize.

The future of aging is not about chasing immortality – it's about preserving energy and vitality. While some of these therapies may take time to become widely available, their message is clear: science is on your side. We're learning more each day about how to slow, even reverse, aspects of aging that once felt inevitable. So stay curious. Stay open. And while you wait for these breakthroughs to mature, remember – you already have powerful tools at your fingertips: nourishing food, movement, sleep, stress relief, and meaningful connection. Longevity isn't a distant dream – it's a daily choice, available to you right now.

CHAPTER 10:
ETHICAL AND CULTURAL CONSIDERATIONS AND THE FUTURE OF HUMAN LONGEVITY

"Just because we can extend life doesn't mean we should – until we understand how to do it with purpose."

— Maria L. Ellis, BBA, MBA

Elena had always lived simply. A retired nurse living in a modest apartment in Queens, she spent her days volunteering at the local community center, helping seniors navigate health insurance paperwork and offering comfort to those newly diagnosed with chronic conditions. At seventy-six, her body ached more than it used to, but her mind was sharp and her spirit generous. She didn't dream of living to 120 – she just wanted to stay independent, stay useful, and stay close to her grandkids.

One afternoon, after watching a documentary about a billionaire tech entrepreneur pursuing "biological immortality," Elena laughed, turned to me, and said, "So now you need a few million just to age gracefully?" It was a joke, but there was a deep truth in her voice. She had watched health and wellness evolve from vitamins and superfoods to stem cells and gene therapy. While she admired the science, she also saw how quickly it could create distance between those who could access these innovations and those who could not.

Her words stayed with me. Because while we celebrate the breakthroughs in longevity science – and we should – we also have to ask: Who gets to benefit? What values are we promoting? And are we creating a future that's not only longer, but also fairer?

That's what this chapter is about.

We'll explore the ethical questions that arise as life-extending technologies become more advanced – and more expensive. We'll look at cultural attitudes around aging, how privilege can shape access to longevity, and whether the pursuit of youth is leaving behind the very people who need care the most. We'll also unpack the role of health influencers and the growing conversation around biohacking – what's helpful, what's hype, and where we draw the line between innovation and obsession.

Because longevity isn't just a personal choice – it's a societal one. And how we move forward matters.

What This Means to You

Elena's story reminds us that the future of longevity must be guided by compassion, accessibility, and shared humanity. As you think about your longevity journey, ask yourself not only how long you want to live, but how you can contribute to a world where others have the opportunity to thrive as well. Supporting equitable healthcare, staying informed, and advocating for inclusive innovation are ways each of us can make a difference. True longevity is not just about extending life – it's about expanding dignity, purpose, and opportunity for everyone.

The Ethics of Living Longer

Scientific breakthroughs in longevity are already triggering urgent ethical dilemmas. Should everyone have access to life-extending treatments? What impact will extreme longevity have on society, the economy, and natural resources? This chapter explores the moral, social, and philosophical questions surrounding human lifespan extension, featuring real-world stories of individuals grappling with these issues.

The pursuit of human longevity has entered uncharted territory. With breakthroughs in genetic engineering, regenerative medicine, and AI-driven health optimization, we are no longer simply prolonging life – we are redefining what it means to age.

But as science pushes the limits of lifespan extension, it also raises profound ethical dilemmas: Should extreme longevity be a privilege for the wealthy, or a right for all? How will extended lifespans impact global resources, the economy, and population dynamics? Will we redefine what it means to "age" and "die," or will we create new societal divides? These are no longer hypotheticals – they're real-world challenges we must confront together.

This chapter explores the moral, social, and philosophical questions surrounding lifespan extension, featuring real-world stories of individuals, scientists, and ethicists grappling with these dilemmas. From the billionaires investing in immortality to the global leaders navigating the societal impact, the future of longevity is more than just science – it is a question of purpose, fairness, and the kind of world we want to create. Living longer is no longer just a possibility – it's an ethical decision. The future of human longevity demands that we not only ask how far we can go, but also why, for whom, and at what cost.

Ethical Dilemmas in Longevity Science

The Question of Access: Who Gets to Live Longer?

One of the biggest concerns in longevity science is equal access. Cutting-edge treatments like gene therapy, stem cell rejuvenation, and AI-driven care are prohibitively expensive, raising fears they'll serve only the wealthy.

Should life-extending treatments be considered a human right or a privilege? How can we ensure these breakthroughs are accessible to all, not just the elite?

Story: Elena's Dilemma: The Price of Extended Life

At seventy-eight years old, Elena had lived a fulfilling life as a beloved teacher, mentor, and lifelong learner. She had shaped countless young minds, instilled a love of literature in her students, and left a lasting mark on her community. But as she aged, she began to feel the weight of time on her body – her joints ached, her energy waned, and she longed for the vitality she once had.

Then, one day, she read about a revolutionary new stem cell treatment – a breakthrough that promised to regenerate aging tissues, restore mobility, and even reverse some of the biological damage of aging. The science was compelling, the testimonials inspiring. For the first time, living longer didn't just seem like a dream – it felt possible.

But when she looked at the price tag, her heart sank. $100,000 for a full course of therapy.

For some, that might be a small investment. But for Elena, a retired teacher on a fixed income, it was an impossible sum. She spent her life educating others, yet now faced a harsh reality.

She wrestled with a difficult question: Would society divide into those who could buy extra decades of life – and those who couldn't?

Would longevity treatments become a privilege for the elite, leaving everyone else to age in the shadows of those who could pay for youth?

As she sat in her cozy reading nook, surrounded by books filled with centuries of human wisdom, she pondered, "If we unlock the secrets of longevity, how do we ensure that those discoveries benefit all of humanity – not just the wealthy few?"

Elena's story is a reflection of one of the biggest ethical

dilemmas of modern longevity science. As life-extending therapies become a reality, will access be based on need or net worth? Will these innovations empower society as a whole or deepen social inequality?

Her question remained unanswered, but one truth was clear: the future of longevity must be driven not just by science, but by justice.

Overpopulation and Resource Scarcity: The Price of Longer Lives

The dream of living to 120 and beyond is becoming more plausible with advancements in genetics, regenerative medicine, and AI-driven healthcare. But with longer lifespans come urgent questions: Can the planet sustain a growing population where people live for an extra fifty years? How will we manage food, water, and energy demands in a world where lifespans are doubled? Will housing shortages skyrocket, forcing societies to rethink urban planning and sustainability? How will retirement, employment, and social security systems adjust if people remain in the workforce for decades longer?

Governments and policymakers will be forced to confront complex, paradigm-shifting challenges as the traditional life cycle – education, work, retirement – becomes obsolete. Will increased longevity overpopulate the Earth, or will declining birth rates naturally counterbalance extended lifespans?

Story: John's Vision – Reimagining Society for a World Without Aging

John, a pioneering longevity scientist, doesn't just study aging – he believes in a future where it's optional. He envisions a world where science doesn't just extend life but enhances it, creating a society that thrives economically, socially, and ecologically in the face of radical longevity. Instead of fearing overpopulation, John sees opportunity. He advocates for sustainability initiatives – investments in vertical farming, lab-grown meat, renewable energy, and water conservation to meet the demands of a growing, long-lived population. Workforce adaptation – redesigning careers and education, enabling people to reskill, transition industries, and remain productive well into their centenarian years rather than retiring at sixty-five. AI and automation integration – using artificial intelligence and robotics to support human longevity, ensuring longer lives don't lead to increased economic strain but rather to greater efficiency, innovation, and quality of life.

John believes that longevity science isn't just about adding years to life – it's about rethinking society from the ground up. To him, aging is a technical problem, not an inevitability, and its elimination should be met with intelligent, ethical solutions that ensure the world doesn't just survive longer lifespans – it thrives with them. Longer lives demand smarter societies. The future of longevity will require bold innovation, sustainable resource management, and radical policy shifts to ensure that life extension benefits all of humanity – without depleting the planet that sustains us.

The Philosophical Debate: Should We Extend Life at All?

As science pushes the boundaries of human lifespan, a profound question emerges: Just because we can extend life, should we? Does extending life indefinitely rob it of significance? Would immortality strip away the urgency that gives life its meaning? How do we balance longevity with purpose, wisdom, and fulfillment?

For some, the pursuit of longevity is an extraordinary opportunity – a chance to see future generations flourish, to continue contributing to society, and to experience more of the world's beauty. But for others, aging is a natural part of life's cycle, and attempting to outrun mortality raises deep ethical, cultural, and philosophical concerns.

Many religious, spiritual, and philosophical traditions

teach that mortality is essential to human experience – that the awareness of death gives life urgency, shapes our decisions, and drives us to find meaning in our limited time. Without an endpoint, do our choices lose weight? Does a limitless life become less rich, less valuable?

Story: Jenny's Reflection – The Soul of Longevity

At ninety years old, Jenny had witnessed a lifetime of change, love, and loss. She had seen the birth of her grandchildren, the passing of dear friends, the evolution of society before her eyes. She cherished life's vibrancy, but reading about new longevity therapies – from gene editing to organ regeneration – stirred a mix of hope and unease. She loved life, yes. But she wondered: Would living decades longer make life fuller, or would it dilute the richness of experience?

If death were no longer inevitable, would we still live with urgency – or drift without direction?

Jenny pondered the wisdom of generations before her – philosophers, poets, and thinkers who had all wrestled with the reality of mortality. She realized that while medical advancements might extend life, true longevity isn't about more years – it's about making those years matter. For her, the question was no longer simply "How long can we live?" but rather, "How do we live in a way that makes extended time truly worthwhile?"

The Purpose of Longevity

Longevity without purpose is merely existence. As we move closer to the possibility of radically extended lifespans, we must also cultivate wisdom, emotional well-being, and spiritual fulfillment to ensure that longer lives are not just longer – but richer, deeper, and more meaningful.

The Future of Human Longevity: Finding a Balanced Approach

While the future of longevity is filled with promise, responsible and ethical implementation is key. Governments, scientists, and ethicists must work together to ensure longer lives are also fulfilling, equitable, and sustainable.

The pursuit of extending human lifespan has transitioned from the realm of science fiction to a tangible scientific endeavor. Advancements in biotechnology, medicine, and a deeper understanding of the aging process have propelled life extension research to the forefront of scientific discourse. However, as we venture into this promising territory, it is imperative to address the ethical, social, and economic dimensions that accompany the quest for prolonged vitality.

The Imperative of Transparency in Life Extension Research

Transparency is the cornerstone of ethical, trustworthy science. In the context of life extension, openness in research methodologies, funding sources, and potential conflicts of interest is crucial for several reasons:

- Building Public Trust: Historically, life extension research has faced skepticism due to ethical controversies and overhyped claims. Transparent practices can rebuild public confidence by demonstrating integrity and accountability.
- Facilitating Collaborative Progress: Open sharing of data and findings accelerates scientific progress by allowing researchers worldwide to build upon each other's work, fostering innovation and avoiding redundant efforts.
- Ensuring Ethical Integrity: Transparency in clinical trials and experimental procedures ensures adherence to ethical standards, safeguarding participant welfare and upholding human rights.

Prioritizing Affordability in Life Extension Interventions

As life-extending therapies emerge, ensuring their affordability is essential to prevent exacerbating social inequalities. High costs can limit access to advanced treatments, leading to a disparity where only affluent individuals benefit from longevity advancements. Affordable interventions can improve public health, reduce age-related disease burdens, and ease strain on healthcare systems. Making these treatments accessible is key to long-term economic stability.

Case Study: The Economic Implications of Healthcare Affordability – A Billion-Dollar Key to Longevity

Access to quality healthcare is not just a moral issue – it's an economic one. As the cost of medical treatments, prescriptions, and emerging life-extension therapies continues to soar, millions are left wondering: Will longevity be reserved for the wealthy, or will it become an accessible reality for all? A groundbreaking report by PatientRightsAdvocate.org sheds light on a staggering truth – lack of healthcare price transparency is one of the biggest barriers to affordability, driving up costs, limiting access, and ultimately shortening lifespans.

What This Means to You

The rising cost of healthcare and the lack of price transparency impact more than just your wallet – they can determine your access to the treatments and preventive care that support a longer, healthier life. As you plan your personal longevity journey, it's essential to be proactive: ask for clear pricing information, advocate for fair healthcare practices, and seek providers who prioritize transparency. Recognizing that affordability is a critical pillar of true longevity empowers you to make informed choices, demand accountability, and contribute to a future where extended life isn't a privilege reserved for the few, but a right accessible to all.

The Report's Key Findings: The Financial Impact of Transparency

Over $1 Trillion in Potential Savings – The report revealed that enforcing healthcare price transparency – ensuring that hospitals and insurers disclose real costs – could slash national healthcare spending by over $1 trillion annually. Longer, Healthier Lives – When people can afford preventive care, early interventions, and emerging longevity treatments, they experience fewer chronic illnesses, lower rates of medical bankruptcy, and increased life expectancy. Barriers to Healthcare Access = Shortened Lifespans – The current system prioritizes opaque pricing, inflated costs, and hidden fees, preventing millions from seeking life-saving treatments. The result? Delayed care, unmanaged chronic conditions, and preventable deaths.

The Longevity Equation: Affordable Healthcare = Extended Lifespan

The report underscores a critical truth: Economic accessibility is a cornerstone of human longevity. If life-extending therapies – such as stem cell regeneration, gene editing, and AI-driven early disease detection – are priced out of reach for the majority, we risk creating a two-tiered society: one where the wealthy live decades longer while the rest struggle with preventable aging-related diseases.

Healthcare Reform is a Longevity Strategy

The potential to extend life expectancy isn't just locked in scientific breakthroughs – it's tied directly to financial and systemic reforms. By making healthcare pricing transparent and accessible, we can unlock longer, healthier lives for all – not just those who can afford it. Enforcing price transparency can reduce national spending and increase access to life-saving treatments. Affordable preventive care extends lifespans and lowers the burden of chronic diseases, and ensuring equitable access to longevity therapies is a critical step in reshaping the future of aging. Longevity should not be a privilege – it should be a right. True progress in anti-aging and healthcare innovation must be paired with economic reforms that prioritize affordability, transparency, and access for all.

Policy Considerations for Social and Economic Adaptation to Extended Lifespans

Prolonged lifespans necessitate comprehensive policy reforms to address the accompanying social and economic challenges, including Pension System Reforms. Traditional retirement models may become unsustainable. Policies could include adjusting retirement ages and restructuring pension schemes to reflect longer working lives. Healthcare Infrastructure: An aging population requires robust healthcare services focused on geriatric care, chronic disease management, and preventive measures, and Labor Market Adaptations: Encouraging lifelong learning and flexible work arrangements can help older individuals remain productive, benefiting the economy and personal fulfillment.

Case Study: The Role of Social Policies in Health Outcomes – Why Longevity is More Than Just Medicine

When we think of extending human life, we often focus on medical breakthroughs, cutting-edge treatments, and advancements in biotechnology. But what if the key to longevity isn't just in the lab – it's also in the policies that govern our societies?

Research has uncovered a critical yet often overlooked factor: Nations that invest more in social policies – such as education, housing, income security, and community well-being – tend to have higher life expectancy and better overall health outcomes. Conversely, lower social expenditures in the U.S. may be contributing to less favorable trends in life expectancy, despite advances in healthcare.

What This Means to You

The link between social policy and health reminds us: longevity isn't just personal – it's collective. While individual choices – diet, exercise, supplements – are important, advocating for stronger community support systems matters too. As you invest in your personal health, also consider how you can support broader changes that create healthier environments for everyone. A longer, healthier life is not just about what happens inside your body – it's also shaped by the world you help build around you.

The Research Findings: Social Investment = Longer, Healthier Lives

Lower U.S. Life Expectancy Compared to Other Developed Nations – Despite having some of the world's most advanced medical institutions, the U.S. lags behind in life expectancy. Researchers point to weaker social safety nets and economic inequalities as contributing factors. Health is More Than Just Healthcare – Countries with robust social policies – such as universal healthcare, paid parental leave, affordable housing, and access to nutritious food – experience lower rates of chronic disease, mental health disorders, and premature death. Stability = Longevity – Individuals with financial security, stable housing, and strong community support experience less stress, lower rates of cardiovascular disease, and improved mental well-being – key factors in longevity.

The Longevity Equation: Social Well-Being is Preventative Medicine

Longevity isn't just about extending lifespan – it's about improving quality of life. Science alone cannot solve the problem of declining life expectancy if people lack access to stable incomes, safe neighborhoods, education, and social support. Countries that prioritize social well-being alongside medical innovation see better public health outcomes, lower healthcare costs, and increased life expectancy.

If we are serious about extending human lifespan, we must think beyond drugs and therapies and look at the bigger picture – how social systems shape health and longevity. Investing in education, social security, and community health leads to longer, healthier lives. Economic security and access to essential services reduce stress and improve well-being, and a society that values social policies as much as medical advancements creates the foundation for lasting longevity. Health doesn't begin in the exam room – it begins in the systems that shape how we live. If we truly want to extend life expectancy, we must invest in people – not just medicine.

A Holistic Approach to Life Extension

The pursuit of life extension transcends scientific breakthroughs; it demands a holistic approach that integrates ethical transparency, economic accessibility, adaptive policies, and the nurturing of personal fulfillment. By embracing this comprehensive perspective, society can ensure that extended lifespans are not only longer but also richer and more meaningful.

Based on my research for Balancing Ethics and Longevity Technologies, consider the New Energy Healing: BioCharger NG, which enhances the body's ability to restore and recover using four scientifically proven energy types: light, PEMF, frequency harmonics, and voltage. Advancements in biotechnology and medicine have brought the possibility of significantly extending human lifespan closer to reality. While the prospect of prolonging life is appealing, it raises complex ethical questions concerning resource allocation, population dynamics, quality of life, and equitable access to life-extending interventions. This chapter delves into these moral considerations, emphasizing the importance of a balanced and inclusive approach to life extension technologies.

Resource Allocation and Societal Impact

The development and implementation of life extension therapies could place substantial demands on healthcare systems. Allocating resources to such interventions may divert attention and funding from addressing existing health disparities and treating acute conditions. Ethicists caution that prioritizing life extension could exacerbate inequalities in healthcare access and outcomes.

Extending human lifespan may have profound economic consequences, including increased pension liabilities, shifts in workforce demographics, and challenges in sustaining social welfare programs. Policymakers must consider how to adapt economic structures to accommodate a population with a significantly prolonged lifespan.

Prolonging life could contribute to overpopulation, intensifying environmental degradation and resource depletion. Critics argue that extending lifespan without addressing birth rates may lead to unsustainable population growth, exacerbating issues such as climate change and habitat loss. Life extension raises questions about fairness between generations. Allocating resources to extend the lives of current generations might limit opportunities and resources available to future generations, potentially leading to intergenerational tensions and ethical dilemmas.

Quality of Life and the Nature of Aging

Extending lifespan without ensuring a corresponding extension of health span – the period of life spent in good health – may result in prolonged periods of morbidity. Ethical considerations must address whether life extension technologies can enhance the quality of life and not merely extend the duration of life. Some philosophers argue that mortality gives meaning to human life, and that extending life indefinitely could alter the human experience in undesirable ways. Concerns include the potential loss of motivation, purpose, and the natural progression of life stages.

Ensuring that life extension interventions are accessible to all, regardless of socioeconomic status, is a significant ethical challenge. Without deliberate policies to promote equity, there is a risk that such technologies could be available only to the affluent, exacerbating existing social inequalities. The global distribution of life extension technologies must be considered, particularly in low- and middle-income countries where basic healthcare needs are still unmet. Ethical frameworks should guide the dissemination of these interventions to prevent widening global health disparities.

Policy Recommendations for Ethical Life Extension

Engaging diverse stakeholders, including ethicists, policymakers, scientists, and the public, in discussions about life extension is crucial. Such discourse can help identify societal values and priorities, guiding ethical decision-making. Developing comprehensive regulatory frameworks can ensure that life extension technologies are safe, effective, and distributed equitably. Policies must address clinical trial ethics, approval pathways, and ongoing oversight after treatments reach the market. Prioritizing investments in health equity can help mitigate disparities in access to life extension interventions. This includes funding for public health initiatives, subsidies for low-income populations, and international aid to support global health efforts. As humanity stands on the brink of potentially transformative life extension technologies, it is imperative to navigate the ethical landscape thoughtfully. Balancing the desire to prolong life with considerations of resource allocation, population dynamics, quality of life, and equitable access will require collaborative efforts and a commitment to social justice. By addressing these ethical challenges proactively, society can strive to ensure that the benefits of life extension are realized responsibly and inclusively.

Cultural Perspectives on Aging and Longevity

Different cultures have unique attitudes and practices related to aging. Exploring these can provide insights into various approaches to longevity and the societal factors that influence aging. A cultural lens offers a holistic view of longevity, encompassing the social, ethical, and technological forces that shape how we age. Aging is a universal human experience, yet perceptions and practices surrounding it vary significantly across cultures. These cultural attitudes profoundly influence how societies approach longevity, elder care, and the value placed on older adults. By examining diverse cultural perspectives, we can gain insights into various approaches to aging and the societal factors that promote longevity.

In many Western societies, aging is often viewed through a lens of decline and loss. The emphasis on youthfulness and productivity can lead to negative stereotypes about older adults. Western culture frequently associates aging with physical decline and diminished social value. This perspective fuels a robust anti-aging industry, with individuals investing in cosmetic procedures, supplements, and fitness regimens to maintain a youthful appearance. Media representations often glorify youth, further entrenching ageist attitudes.

Recent studies indicate a gradual shift in these perceptions. Research published in "Psychology and Aging" found that individuals now perceive old age to begin later than in previous decades, reflecting changing attitudes toward aging and increased longevity.

In contrast, many Eastern cultures hold more reverential views of aging, emphasizing respect for elders and valuing their wisdom. In countries influenced by Confucianism, such as China, Korea, and Japan, filial piety is a core value. This principle dictates a deep respect for one's parents and ancestors, manifesting in practices that honor and care for the elderly. Older adults are often seen as bearers of wisdom and are integral to family and societal decision-making.

Research comparing aging perceptions between Japanese and American adults found that Japanese individuals exhibit more positive aging profiles. This outlook is attributed to cultural norms that value aging and integrate older adults into the community, contributing to their well-being and longevity.

Indigenous cultures often possess unique views on aging, viewing it as a natural and respected phase of life. In many Indigenous communities, elders are revered as custodians of cultural knowledge, traditions, and history. They play a crucial role in educating younger generations and maintaining the cultural fabric of the community. Aging is seen as an accumulation of wisdom and a time for continued contribution. These cultures often emphasize communal living and support, ensuring that older adults are cared for within the community. This collective approach fosters a sense of belonging and purpose among the elderly, which is linked to improved health outcomes and longevity.

The Impact of Cultural Attitudes on Longevity

Cultural perspectives on aging significantly influence health behaviors, policy development, and the overall well-being of older adults. Cultures that value aging and integrate older adults into daily life often promote healthier behaviors. For instance, the Mediterranean lifestyle, prevalent in parts of Europe, emphasizes balanced nutrition, regular physical activity, and strong social connections, all of which contribute to longevity.

Societal attitudes toward aging inform public policies related to elder care, retirement, and healthcare. Cultures that uphold respect for the elderly are more likely to implement supportive policies that enhance the quality of life for older adults, such as accessible healthcare services and social welfare programs.

The Okinawan Approach: Timeless Wisdom for a Longer, Healthier Life

Nestled in the tropical archipelago of Japan, Okinawa is home to one of the highest concentrations of centenarians in the world. Unlike many parts of the globe where aging is associated with decline, Okinawans embody vitality, resilience, and purpose well into their nineties and beyond. Scientists and longevity researchers have spent decades studying what makes Okinawan culture so unique, and the findings reveal a holistic blueprint for longevity – one deeply embedded in lifestyle, mindset, and community.

The Secrets Behind Okinawan Longevity

Ikigai: The Art of Living with Purpose. Okinawans don't retire from life – they lean into it. Ikigai is the Japanese philosophy of "reason for being," a guiding force that keeps people engaged, motivated, and fulfilled. Whether it's tending to a garden, mentoring younger generations, or practicing a lifelong craft, Okinawans wake up each day with a purpose – something greater than themselves. Research links having a strong sense of purpose to lower stress, a reduced risk of cardiovascular disease, and even an extended lifespan. A study found that individuals who embrace their Ikigai live an average of seven years longer than those without a clear life purpose.

Hara Hachi Bu: The Art of Eating Wisely. Unlike the Western habit of eating until completely full, Okinawans follow the Confucian principle of Hara Hachi Bu – eating until they are only 80 percent full. This practice naturally reduces caloric intake, supports digestion, and prevents metabolic disorders associated with overeating. Caloric restriction without malnutrition has been linked to lower oxidative stress, reduced inflammation, and a longer lifespan. Okinawans consume low-calorie, high-nutrient traditional diets rich in vegetables, sweet potatoes, tofu, and seaweed – fueling their bodies with longevity-enhancing nutrients.

Longevity is a Lifestyle, Not Just a Science. The Okinawan approach to aging is a masterclass in holistic wellness. It teaches us that a long, healthy life isn't just about diet and exercise – it's about connection, purpose, and mindful living. Prioritize relationships and create a strong support network. Find your Ikigai – your reason to wake up with joy and intention – and practice mindful eating and caloric moderation for metabolic health. Modern medicine may extend lifespan, but the Okinawan way of life enhances health span. By integrating community, purpose, and balance, we can learn to not only live longer – but live better.

The Sardinian Lifestyle: A Blueprint for Longevity in the Heart of the Mediterranean

Nestled in the azure waters of the Mediterranean, Sardinia, Italy, stands as a beacon of exceptional longevity. This rugged island, home to one of the world's highest concentrations of male centenarians, offers a lifestyle deeply intertwined with nature, family, and tradition. Sardinians don't just live longer – they thrive, embodying vitality and resilience well into their nineties and hundreds. So, what is the secret to Sardinian longevity? Researchers have uncovered a powerful combination of strong family ties, natural movement, and a heart-healthy Mediterranean diet – all of which work together to create a sustainable, joyful, and health-enhancing way of life.

The Pillars of Sardinian Longevity

Strong Family Bonds: A Life Anchored in Love and Purpose

Sardinian culture places immense value on family, respect for elders, and intergenerational living. Unlike in many modern societies, Sardinian elders remain central to family life – sharing wisdom, caregiving, and connection.

Studies have shown that strong social connections can increase lifespan by up to 50 percent. Emotional support from family lowers stress, reduces inflammation, and strengthens the immune system, providing a biological shield against aging-related diseases.

Unlike structured gym workouts, Sardinians stay fit naturally – through daily movement, farming, herding livestock, and walking the island's steep, hilly terrains. This low-intensity, high-frequency physical activity builds strong muscles, maintains cardiovascular health, and prevents metabolic decline. Research on Blue Zones (regions with the highest life expectancy) confirms that consistent, moderate physical activity – even something as simple as walking five miles a day – lowers the risk of heart disease, stroke, and cognitive decline. At the heart of Sardinian health is a traditional, nutrient-rich, plant-based diet. Meals are centered around fresh vegetables, legumes, whole grains, nuts, and extra virgin olive oil, with modest amounts of meat and dairy. Red wine, rich in antioxidants, is often enjoyed in moderation.

Sardinians naturally follow a high-fiber, low-inflammatory diet that protects against heart disease, diabetes, and cancer. Their polyphenol-rich red wine (often homemade) contributes to better circulation and reduced oxidative stress. The Sardinian way of life teaches us that longevity is not just about years – it's about quality of life. They don't chase longevity through science and technology; they live it naturally, through deep relationships, physical movement, and a diet rich in nature's best offerings. Longevity is not a mystery – it's a lifestyle. The Sardinian way of life reminds us that connection, movement, and mindful nutrition are the true elixirs of a long, fulfilling existence.

Embracing Cultural Diversity in Aging

Understanding cultural perspectives on aging offers valuable insights into practices that promote longevity and enhance the quality of life for older adults. By appreciating and integrating diverse cultural attitudes, societies can develop more inclusive and effective approaches to aging, ensuring that the later stages of life are viewed as periods of opportunity, respect, and continued growth. As we move closer to unlocking the secrets of extended life, the challenge is not just how long we live but how well we live. Ethical and cultural considerations must guide advancements, ensuring that longevity benefits all of humanity, not just a select few.

As we stand on the threshold of extraordinary advancements in longevity science, we must remember that how we age – and how we extend life – should reflect not just innovation, but intention. It's not enough to live longer if we don't also live with equity, empathy, and inclusivity. Elena reminds us that dignity, purpose, and human connection matter as much as scientific progress. The true future of longevity must not only ask how long we can live, but also for whom we are making that future possible. Let's ensure that as we pursue progress, we also preserve our humanity.

CHAPTER 11:
INTEGRATING LONGEVITY PRACTICES INTO EVERYDAY LIFE

*"Longevity is not a destination; it's a way
of living, one choice at a time."*
— Maria L. Ellis, BBA, MBA

To celebrate my seventy-fifth birthday, I went to Tuscany, Italy, with a group of dear friends. We rented a charming farmhouse nestled among rolling hills and endless groves of ancient olive trees. Each morning, we gathered on the terrace overlooking the golden fields to practice yoga. The crisp air carried the scent of rosemary and wildflowers, and the soft chirping of birds served as our meditation soundtrack.

Some days, after yoga, we would wander through the olive groves, soaking up the sun and the serene beauty of the land. It became a playful tradition to hug the gnarled, ancient olive trees – a way of grounding ourselves, thanking nature for its timeless wisdom. During this trip, I had also decided to challenge myself by learning how to speak Italian. Every day, I practiced phrases, listened carefully to the locals, and stumbled through conversations with a smile.

One particular afternoon, as I wrapped my arms

around a particularly majestic olive tree, I suddenly felt a tickling sensation crawling up my arms. Laughing and eager to show off my new Italian skills, I turned to my friends and exclaimed, "Questo albero è pieno di aunts!" – accidentally mixing English with Italian. I meant to say ants, but it came out sounding like the tree was full of "aunties."

The image of dozens of little Italian "zie" bustling around the tree set off a wave of uncontrollable laughter among my friends and me. Even as I brushed them off, the joy of that silly moment stayed with me. It was a reminder that learning, laughter, and connection don't end with age – they deepen, becoming the true gifts of a well-lived life. And as the sun set over the rolling Tuscan hills, while I was enjoying an Aperol Spritz that evening, I smiled to myself and whispered, "La vita è bella" – life is beautiful.

What This Means to You

Moments of laughter, connection, and even a little silliness are powerful medicine for the mind and spirit. As we age, it's easy to believe that growth, learning, and pure joy belong to the past – but they are very much a part of a vibrant, healthy future. Hugging olive trees, learning a new language, laughing over mistakes, and sharing experiences with friends are not trivial acts; they are profound investments in emotional resilience, cognitive vitality, and overall longevity.

The lesson is simple: keep seeking new experiences, keep surrounding yourself with people who lift your spirit, and never underestimate the healing power of nature – and a good laugh.

Morning: Fueling Body and Brain

My mornings now begin with intention. I start with a tall glass of lemon water to rehydrate and wake up my system.

Then I stretch, move my body, and enjoy a walk around the block, sometimes listening to Italian audio lessons on my earbuds. Nothing strenuous – just joyful movement to wake me up and get my blood flowing. When I return, I make a nutrient-rich breakfast – usually something with protein, berries, and greens. Because this seventy-five-year-old brain needs fuel to learn new words! And then, I study. Not for hours – just twenty or thirty minutes. I repeat the phrases out loud. I write them down. I stumble, laugh at myself, then try again. It's humbling and exhilarating all at once. "Mi chiamo Maria. Ho settantacinque anni. Studio l'italiano." I speak it like a child – but I do it with pride.

Afternoon: Balance, Boundaries, and Beauty

Midday, I pause for a healthy lunch, sometimes followed by a short rest or a moment of stillness. I protect my energy now – not out of weakness, but wisdom. I check in with friends, write a bit, maybe do a little gardening or review a few flashcards while sitting in the sun. Every part of this rhythm is a longevity practice: sunlight, movement, connection, curiosity.

And most importantly, I say no more often – to unnecessary obligations, to noise, to anything that doesn't align with my values or vitality. Stress isn't something I glamorize anymore. Peace is the new power.

Evening: Reflect, Restore, Rejoice

As the day winds down, I begin my evening ritual – dim lights, herbal tea, no screens. I often journal, writing in both English and, yes, a few lines in Italian. I track what I've learned, how I felt, what energized me. I sleep better now – deep, restorative sleep – because my days are full of purpose, pleasure, and care.

This chapter isn't really about Italian – it's about living fully, expansively, and with intention. It's about saying yes to something that lights you up inside, even when the world expects you to slow down or stay still. This day-in-the-life isn't fiction – it's real. It's mine. And it can be yours, too.

You now have the tools: the nutrition, the movement, the mindset, the science. But the true magic happens when you live it – when you wake up one day and say, "Why not?"

Because you're never too old, too late, or too far behind to begin again.

You are the author of your longevity. And your next chapter can be the most inspiring one yet. Buonanotte, cara amica. Tomorrow is waiting – with open arms and maybe a few Italian verbs.

Making Longevity a Lifestyle

Living a long and healthy life isn't about quick fixes or miracle cures – it's about creating sustainable habits that enhance physical, mental, and emotional well-being. In this chapter, we will explore how to integrate longevity practices into daily routines, providing actionable steps and real-life stories of individuals who have successfully adopted these strategies.

Creating a Longevity-Focused Daily Routine

Drinking a glass of water with lemon and electrolytes rehydrates the body and kickstarts metabolism. Mindfulness and Gratitude – Spending five minutes journaling or meditating sets a positive tone for the day.

Movement Before Screens – A morning walk or stretching session energizes the body and mind.

Instead of reaching for coffee first thing in the morning, I start my day with a warm glass of lemon water – a simple ritual known to hydrate, alkalize, and awaken the body from the inside out. I follow this with a ten-minute stretching routine, incorporating gentle yoga-inspired movements to improve circulation, release muscle stiffness, and stimulate my nervous system. This morning routine makes me feel more alert, my digestion improved, and my energy lasts longer throughout the day. Instead of the caffeine rollercoaster, I always have sustained, natural energy that helps me focus, move with ease, and feel lighter both physically and mentally.

The Science behind my morning ritual. Warm Lemon Water for Hydration and Detoxification – After seven to eight hours of sleep, the body is dehydrated. Lemon water kickstarts digestion, balances pH levels, and supports liver function, providing gentle, natural wakefulness without caffeine jitters. Stretching for Circulation and Mobility – Morning movement increases blood flow, lubricates joints, and wakes up the nervous system, signaling to the body that it's time to be alert and energized. By nourishing my body before consuming coffee, I prevent adrenal fatigue and energy crashes, leading to a more sustained and balanced sense of alertness. Energy isn't just about caffeine – it's about how you start your day. A simple shift in morning habits can set the tone for vitality, mental clarity, and overall well-being. Longevity isn't about adding years – it's about infusing each day with energy and meaning. My morning ritual is a powerful reminder that small, mindful changes can unlock a more vibrant, energized life.

Optimizing Nutrition and Eating Habits

Time-Restricted Eating – Following a twelve- to sixteen-hour fasting window supports metabolic flexibility and cellular repair. Nutrient-Dense Meals – Prioritizing lean proteins, healthy fats, and fiber-rich vegetables fuels the body efficiently.

Supplementation – Taking essential nutrients like Omega-3s, Vitamin D, and probiotics supports longevity.

My Metabolic Reset at Seventy-Five: A Journey to Renewed Energy and Vitality

At seventy-five years old, I found myself facing a frustrating reality: unwanted weight gain, erratic blood sugar levels, and an increasing reliance on diabetes medication. No matter how carefully I ate or how much I tried to stay active, my metabolism felt sluggish, unresponsive, and out of sync with my body's needs. For years, I believed that aging naturally meant a slower metabolism, more medications, and less control over my health – until I discovered a powerful metabolic reset that changed everything.

My Turning Point: Intermittent Fasting and Eliminating Processed Sugar. After diving into research on longevity and metabolic health, I made two simple but profound changes: Intermittent Fasting – Instead of eating throughout the day, I adopted a 16:8 fasting routine, giving my body more time to rest, repair, and regulate blood sugar naturally. Also, I eliminated refined sugars and ultra-processed foods, replacing them with whole, nutrient-dense meals that stabilized my energy and supported my metabolism.

If you're struggling with weight, blood sugar issues, or metabolic slowdowns, know that your body is capable of change – at any age. Aging doesn't mean surrendering to metabolic decline. With the right approach, you can reset, rebuild, and rediscover the energy, clarity, and vitality that your body is capable of – no matter your age.

Movement and Strength Training for Longevity

Longevity isn't just about adding years to your life – it's about adding life to your years. The key to staying strong, mobile, and independent well into old age lies in daily movement, strength training, and flexibility work. Science shows that staying physically active isn't just about fitness – it's a powerful tool to slow aging, enhance cognitive function, and prevent chronic disease.

Here are some of my simple yet powerful longevity habits.

Walking. I love walking on the beach either at sunrise or sunset. Walking is one of the most underrated yet effective forms of movement. It keeps the heart strong, metabolism active, and circulation flowing, while also supporting joint health and mental clarity. Aim for at least 10,000 steps per day to reduce the risk of cardiovascular disease and metabolic disorders. Brisk walking enhances brain function by increasing blood flow and oxygen to the brain, reducing the risk of cognitive decline. Outdoor walking provides fresh air, vitamin D, and stress relief, further boosting longevity benefits.

Resistance Training: The Anti-Aging Secret. Age-related muscle loss, or sarcopenia, is a major health risk – but it's preventable through regular strength training. By incorporating resistance exercises, you preserve muscle mass, support bone density, and maintain metabolic efficiency. Strength training two to three times per week helps build lean muscle, improve insulin sensitivity, and protect against frailty. Bodyweight exercises (push-ups, squats, lunges) or weightlifting enhance mobility, strength, and balance. Stronger muscles mean a stronger metabolism – helping maintain a healthy weight and energy levels as you age.

Recovery and Flexibility: Keeping the Body Agile and Pain-Free. Longevity isn't just about strength – it's about moving with ease and preventing injury. Stretching, yoga, and mobility work increase flexibility, reduce stiffness, and improve posture, ensuring that you stay agile and active well into your later years.

Aging well isn't about extreme fitness – it's about consistency, variety, and listening to your body. Movement isn't just exercise – it's an investment in your future self. The more you move today, the stronger, healthier, and more independent you'll remain for decades to come.

Sleep and Recovery Practices: Unlocking the Power of Rest for Longevity

Sleep isn't just rest – it's renewal. Every night, your body undergoes cellular repair, hormone regulation, and brain detoxification, making quality sleep one of the most powerful anti-aging tools available. Inadequate sleep accelerates aging, impairs immunity, and heightens the risk of chronic illness. But by adopting intentional sleep and recovery habits, you can optimize longevity, enhance cognitive function, and wake up feeling truly refreshed.

The Pillars of Restorative Sleep

Consistent Sleep Schedule: Aligning with Your Circadian Rhythm. Your body thrives on predictability. I go to bed at ten p.m. and wake up at six-thirty a.m., the same time every day – yes, even on weekends – to strengthen my circadian rhythm, improve sleep quality, and boost my energy levels. I like to watch the sunrise most every day, exposing myself to natural light in the morning to reinforce my internal clock and promote alertness. I often avoid late-night meals and caffeine to prevent disruptions in my melatonin production.

Blue Light Management: Protecting Your Natural Sleep Hormones. Screens and artificial lighting emit blue light, which disrupts melatonin production, tricking your brain into thinking it's still daytime. This leads to difficulty falling asleep, shallow rest, and grogginess in the morning. Use blue-light-blocking glasses in the evening to reduce exposure from screens. Switch to dim, warm lighting (like salt lamps or red-hued bulbs) at night to promote relaxation. Enable night mode on devices or avoid screens at least an hour before bed.

My nighttime rituals help signal to my body that it's time to relax and restore. Creating a calming pre-sleep routine helps slow down your nervous system, reduce stress, and prepare the mind for deep rest. I like to read books, meditate, or practice deep slow breathing to activate my parasympathetic nervous system, reducing cortisol (the stress hormone). I love aromatherapy with lavender or chamomile essential oils to help me create a soothing sleep environment.

Sleep is the Ultimate Longevity Hack. Your body heals

while you sleep. Prioritizing rest is just as crucial as diet and exercise in slowing aging, boosting brain function, and ensuring overall vitality. Sleep isn't wasted time – it's an investment in a longer, healthier life. By mastering your sleep habits, you unlock higher energy, sharper thinking, and the power to age gracefully.

Mental and Emotional Longevity

Engaging in new skills, hobbies, and intellectual challenges strengthens cognitive function.

Also, regular interactions with loved ones enhance emotional well-being and longevity.

For mindfulness and stress reduction – Practice meditation, deep breathing, and gratitude to reduce cortisol levels.

My Passion for Languages: A New Chapter at Seventy-Five

At seventy-five years old, I started learning Italian. While some might think language learning is for the young, I saw it as a way to challenge my mind, expand my world, and embrace lifelong curiosity.

What started as a simple desire to speak the language of art, history, and romance quickly became a journey of self-discovery, mental agility, and new friendships.

From the first moment I whispered "Buongiorno" to myself, I felt something ignite within me. Each lesson, each new word was like a puzzle unlocking a hidden part of my brain. Studies have shown that learning a new language can slow cognitive decline, enhance memory, and strengthen neural pathways – and I was living proof of that.

Through an online language group, I connected with like-minded individuals from around the world – people of all ages, all backgrounds, all sharing a love for learning. At any age, we can rewrite our stories. Whether it's a new language, a new hobby, or a new passion, the mind and heart are always ready to embrace something extraordinary. My journey with Italian reminded me that learning is not just about knowledge – it's about joy, connection, and the endless possibilities of life.

Final Thoughts: A Lifetime of Small Changes

Longevity is not about drastic transformations – it's about small, consistent choices that add up over time. By incorporating these strategies into daily life, we can enhance vitality, resilience, and fulfillment well into our later years.

You don't need to spend millions or chase immortality to live fully. You simply need the courage to stay curious, the willingness to care for your body and mind, and the heart to keep dreaming – at any age. Whether it's learning a new language, dancing in your kitchen, or walking a little farther than yesterday, longevity is built one meaningful choice at a time. This story – this glimpse into a day – isn't just mine. It's an invitation for you to imagine what's possible. To reimagine what aging can feel like. To craft a life that nourishes and excites you. And to remember that every day you wake up is another chance to say: I'm still becoming.

The best is not behind you. It's ahead – waiting for you to live it.

CHAPTER 12:
THE FUTURE OF PERSONALIZED LONGEVITY AND AI-DRIVEN HEALTH OPTIMIZATION

"The next revolution in health is not just about living longer, but living smarter."
— Maria L. Ellis, BBA, MBA

The Promise of Personalized Longevity

Imagine waking up and receiving a message from your digital health advisor – an AI-powered assistant that has tracked your sleep, your mood, your stress levels, and your gut microbiome. It suggests a protein-rich breakfast to stabilize your blood sugar, reminds you to stretch before your afternoon meeting, and prompts you to take a twenty-minute walk when your energy dips. Not because it's guessing, but because it knows you – your rhythms, your genetic markers, your habits. It understands how your body ages – and how to slow that process down.

That's not science fiction. That's where we're headed – and it's happening faster than most people realize.

For decades, health advice has been generalized: eat this, move that way, sleep seven to eight hours. But what works for one person may not work for another. Enter the era of personalized, AI-driven longevity – a new frontier where cutting-edge diagnostics, machine learning, and bio-data come together to tailor your health journey down to the molecule.

We're no longer asking, 'What works?' We're asking, 'What works for me?'

Real People, Real Results

The real power of personalized health isn't just in the data – it's in the stories.

Emily, once burned out and inflamed, didn't just find relief through rest and mindfulness. Her transformation accelerated when her wearable device began tracking her stress biomarkers in real time. A simple vibration on her wrist would remind her to pause, breathe, and reset her nervous system – turning reactive living into responsive, conscious care.

David, sixty-eight, had struggled with sleep for years. Generic advice helped a little, but it wasn't until he underwent an at-home epigenetic test and used AI sleep tracking that he discovered his cortisol was peaking late at night due to an undiagnosed sensitivity to blue light. A customized evening light filter and nutrient protocol finally gave him the deep sleep he hadn't had in a decade.

Lisa, fifty-nine, wanted to stay active but was plagued by joint pain and inflammation. A personalized gut health panel revealed specific food intolerances that were silently fueling her discomfort. Within weeks of adjusting her diet, guided by AI-generated recommendations, she was back to hiking trails and doing yoga with joy.

And Mark, seventy-three, had early signs of cognitive decline. Instead of waiting for it to worsen, he leaned into a personalized brain-training and nootropic protocol developed through his AI health coach. Now, he's not only stable – he's thriving. He writes poetry again.

These aren't miracle stories – they're what happens

when technology meets intention, and someone chooses to participate in their own health story.

Tools, Tech, and What to Watch

So what's actually powering this shift?

Here are key AI-powered longevity tools not just on the horizon – but already arriving in homes.

Smart wearables: Modern devices now track far more than steps – including sleep quality, oxygen levels, and stress signals.

They analyze sleep stages, heart rate variability, oxygen levels, and even emotional states through biometric feedback. Tomorrow's wearables will coach you in real time – adjusting your habits on the fly.

Epigenetic testing and AI diagnostics: These at-home kits decode how your lifestyle is influencing your gene expression. Paired with AI, the data becomes actionable – suggesting specific foods, exercise types, and supplements to improve gene-level resilience.

Digital twins and health forecasting: Some companies now build AI models of your body – digital versions that run simulations to test how your body might respond to different treatments, therapies, or even environments. It's like having a virtual you making the mistakes so the real you doesn't have to.

Robotics and assisted longevity: From robotic exoskeletons that support mobility to AI caregivers for the elderly, we're entering a world where technology doesn't just support aging – it elevates it.

Mental health tech: AI companions and virtual therapists are learning how to support emotional wellness, which we now know is directly tied to aging outcomes. Longevity isn't just physical – it's deeply emotional.

The Takeaway

What does all of this mean for you?

The future of health isn't one-size-fits-all – it's hyper-personalized and deeply intentional. And while not every tool is accessible to everyone yet, the trends are clear: longevity will increasingly be about proactive care, guided by technology that knows how to listen to your unique body.

It also means that the real promise of AI and personalization is not just to add years to your life – but to give you more life in your years. More presence. More clarity. More capacity to live the way you want to.

You are not a statistic. You are a story. And with every new breakthrough, that story has more pages to be written – vibrantly, intentionally, and beautifully your own.

The Next Evolution in Longevity Science

We are standing on the edge of a health revolution – one where aging is no longer a passive process but a dynamic, personalized journey. Thanks to artificial intelligence (AI), biotechnology, and precision medicine, we now have the ability to decode, optimize, and extend human health like never before.

Imagine a future where:

AI-driven diagnostics detect diseases years before symptoms appear, allowing for proactive, rather than reactive, treatments.

Gene-editing therapies reverse cellular damage, slowing or even halting the aging process at its root. Wearable biosensors track real-time biomarkers, offering hyper-personalized nutrition, fitness, and lifestyle recommendations tailored to your unique genetic blueprint.

Biohacking tools and regenerative medicine help restore youthful vitality, keeping individuals stronger, sharper, and more resilient well into old age. This is no longer science fiction – it's the new frontier of longevity science. Researchers, tech innovators, and medical pioneers are rewriting the rules of aging, transforming it from an inevitable decline into a well-managed, data-driven process where health and longevity are optimized in real time.

In this chapter, we will explore the latest breakthroughs

in AI-driven longevity research – from deep-learning algorithms that predict disease to AI-powered drug discovery.

The rise of predictive medicine – how cutting-edge diagnostics and digital twin technology are allowing us to customize health interventions like never before.

Real-life stories of individuals already benefiting from AI-driven health optimization, proving that the future of longevity isn't just coming – it's already here.

The future of health isn't just about adding years to life – it's about adding quality, intelligence, and optimization to those years. With AI and precision medicine leading the charge, we are entering an era where living longer and living smarter go hand in hand.

Emily's AI-Guided Anti-Aging Protocol: Rewiring Aging with Smart Technology

At seventy-one years old, Emily had always embraced an active lifestyle, but she couldn't ignore the subtle signs of aging creeping in – slower recovery, persistent fatigue, and changes in her skin's elasticity. She had tried countless diets, supplements, and exercise routines, but the results were inconsistent. Was she missing something?

Then, she discovered an AI-powered longevity concierge service – a cutting-edge system designed to analyze real-time biomarkers, optimize health decisions, and personalize every aspect of wellness based on her unique biological profile. It was like having a futuristic health coach tailored specifically for her DNA.

How AI Transformed Emily's Longevity Strategy

Through wearable biosensors and at-home blood tests, the AI system tracked inflammatory markers, sleep quality, metabolic function, and hormone levels in real time. Instead of generic vitamin regimens, AI curated a hyper-personalized protocol, adjusting her micronutrient intake, hydration, and intermittent fasting windows to match her biological rhythms. The optimized exercise routine analyzed her muscle recovery times and heart rate variability, tailoring her workouts to maximize strength and endurance while minimizing inflammation. AI recommended peptide therapy and red light treatments, improving her collagen production, reducing stiffness, and giving her skin a natural, youthful glow.

The Results: A Decade Reversed

Within months, Emily felt like a new person. She no longer needed afternoon naps or extra caffeine to stay alert. Her joint pain disappeared, and she moved with greater ease.

Her glowing skin and vibrant hair drew compliments on her renewed, youthful appearance. Emily felt more focused, engaged, and mentally clear than she had in years. What amazed her most? The sense of control she regained over her own aging process. Instead of guessing what worked, she had data-driven insights tailored to her unique biology.

The Future of Longevity is Personalized

Emily's journey proves that aging is no longer something we must accept passively. With AI-driven health optimization, we now have the tools to adjust, enhance, and extend our vitality in ways that were unimaginable just a decade ago. Emily didn't just slow aging – she reprogrammed it. With AI as her guide, she is not just living longer – she's living better, stronger, and more vibrantly than ever before.

How AI and Data-Driven Medicine Are Transforming Longevity

AI-powered wearable devices enable real-time tracking of health metrics, providing personalized insights into sleep patterns, heart health, metabolism, and more.

I use Continuous Glucose Monitors (CGMs) like the Freestyle Libre to track my blood sugar fluctuations in real time, helping me tailor my diets for optimal metabolic health.

AI-Driven Sleep Trackers – The Oura Ring and WHOOP band provide insights into sleep cycles, helping users optimize rest and recovery.

Personalized Fitness Recommendations – AI platforms analyze movement data and suggest customized exercise routines for longevity.

David's AI-Enhanced Health Plan: Rewriting the Rules of Aging

At seventy years old, David had always considered himself relatively healthy, but he couldn't ignore the subtle signs of decline – low energy, stubborn inflammation, and workouts that left him feeling more drained than revitalized. He had tried different diets, supplements, and fitness routines over the years, but nothing seemed to work consistently.

That all changed when he discovered an AI-driven health optimization app – a futuristic wellness companion designed to analyze real-time biomarkers, track lifestyle habits, and provide hyper-personalized recommendations for longevity and peak performance.

How AI Transformed David's Health Strategy

By leveraging the following AI-driven health app that tracked his biomarkers, personalized his nutrition, and optimized his exercise routine, David transformed his energy levels, reduced inflammation, and achieved peak physical health beyond what traditional medicine had offered.

Advanced Health Analytics – The app synced with wearable devices to track his sleep quality, heart rate variability, stress levels, and metabolic efficiency. It provided deep insights into his body's needs in ways traditional medicine never had.

Precision Nutrition and Inflammation Control – Instead of following generic diet plans, the AI suggested food choices tailored to his gut microbiome and genetic predispositions, eliminating triggers that had unknowingly caused inflammation for years.

Optimized Exercise Routine – The app analyzed his recovery patterns and designed a strength and endurance regimen that maximized muscle retention and joint health without overexertion.

Sleep Optimization for Cellular Repair – By identifying patterns in his sleep cycles and circadian rhythm, the AI helped him adjust his bedtime, evening light exposure, and melatonin production for deep, restorative sleep.

The Results: A New Lease on Life

Within a few months, David felt like he had reversed years of aging. He no longer felt sluggish in the afternoons. His joints felt stronger, his movement easier, and the brain fog that once clouded his thinking disappeared. He optimized his workouts for muscle gain and metabolic health. For the first time in years, David felt in complete control of his well-being. Instead of blindly experimenting with health trends, he had AI guiding him with real-time, data-driven decisions.

The Takeaway: AI is the Future of Personalized Longevity

David's journey proves that aging no longer has to be a guessing game. AI-driven health tools are empowering individuals to optimize every aspect of their well-being, from metabolism to recovery, with precision. David didn't just get healthier – he redefined what aging means. With AI as his wellness companion, he's living proof that seventy can feel like fifty, and the future of longevity is already here.

Genetic Testing and Precision Medicine

The following advances in genetic sequencing allow for highly personalized health interventions based on an individual's DNA.

Epigenetic Testing – AI can analyze how genes are expressed over time, allowing for tailored anti-aging strategies. Nutrigenomics – Personalized diet plans based on genetic predispositions help prevent diseases before they develop. AI-Guided Drug Development – AI is accelerating the creation of anti-aging compounds and targeted treatments.

Lisa's Genetic Breakthrough: Rewriting Her Brain's Future with AI-Driven Precision

At sixty-eight years old, Lisa had always been sharp, inquisitive, and passionate about learning. But when she took a DNA test out of curiosity, she uncovered something unexpected – a genetic predisposition to early cognitive decline. The results were sobering, a glimpse into a future she wasn't ready to accept.

Instead of resigning herself to fate, Lisa took control – using AI-driven health optimization to create a personalized brain-health strategy designed to slow cognitive aging and enhance her mental agility.

How AI Helped Lisa Protect and Strengthen Her Mind

By leveraging the following AI-driven health insights, Lisa implemented a personalized brain-health strategy – including precision nutrition, cognitive training, targeted supplementation, and optimized sleep – allowing her to slow cognitive decline, enhance mental clarity, and protect her long-term brain function.

Advanced Cognitive Risk Analysis – AI identified key genetic markers linked to cognitive decline and cross-referenced them with lifestyle factors, diet, and environmental influences to create a customized intervention plan. Brain-Boosting Nutrition – Instead of a generic "healthy diet," Lisa received a precision-tailored eating plan designed to reduce neuroinflammation and support neurotransmitter function. She added omega-3s, polyphenols, and MCT oil to her diet – nourishing her brain on a cellular level. Cognitive Training and Neuroplasticity Exercises – AI recommended interactive brain games, memory exercises, and meditation techniques to stimulate neural connections and enhance brain plasticity.

Precision Supplementation – Based on her genetic profile, AI suggested specific nootropic supplements like lion's mane mushroom, resveratrol, and phosphatidylserine to boost cognitive function and protect against neurodegeneration. Optimized Sleep and Stress Reduction – Since poor sleep accelerates brain aging, Lisa followed AI-guided sleep tracking and stress management techniques, ensuring her brain had the recovery time it needed to function at its peak.

The Results: A Sharper Mind, A Brighter Future

Within six months, Lisa felt a profound shift: improved memory recall – she no longer struggled to find the right words or remember small details; sharper focus and mental clarity – she felt more present, engaged, and mentally energized; reduced brain fog and increased processing speed, allowing her to think and react faster; greater confidence in her long-term cognitive health, knowing she was taking proactive steps toward a brighter, stronger future.

Your Genetics Are Not Your Destiny

Lisa's story is a powerful testament to how AI-driven, personalized health strategies can reshape our future – even when genetics seem to suggest otherwise. Lisa didn't accept her genetic fate – she revised the script. With the power of AI, precision medicine, and brain-boosting lifestyle strategies, she's living proof that longevity isn't just about living longer – it's about staying mentally sharp, vibrant, and engaged for decades to come.

AI in Predictive Medicine: Preventing Illness Be-

fore It Starts

AI in predictive medicine is revolutionizing healthcare by enabling early disease detection and prevention through advanced data analysis, improving cancer screening accuracy, predicting cardiovascular risks, and optimizing gut health for enhanced overall well-being. Predictive AI is allowing physicians to identify and treat diseases before symptoms appear by analyzing vast amounts of health data. Cancer Detection – AI is improving early cancer screening, detecting tumors in imaging scans with greater accuracy than human doctors. Heart Disease Prevention – AI-powered algorithms predict cardiovascular risks based on blood pressure, cholesterol, and lifestyle data. AI-Driven Gut Health Analysis – Microbiome testing can optimize digestion, immunity, and overall health.

Mark's AI-Powered Health Transformation: A Life Saved Before a Crisis Began

At seventy-four years old, Mark considered himself in fairly good shape, but deep down, he knew something was off. He often felt fatigued, short of breath, and unusually stressed, yet routine check-ups never flagged anything serious. What if his body was signaling something his doctors weren't seeing yet?

That's when he discovered an AI-driven health optimization program – a revolutionary system that analyzed thousands of biomarkers, genetic data, and lifestyle factors to detect early warning signs of disease long before symptoms appeared.

How AI Uncovered the Silent Danger

Early Heart Disease Detection – AI algorithms identified subtle warning signs in Mark's blood pressure trends, cholesterol ratios, and inflammatory markers, predicting that he was at high risk for a future heart attack – despite having no outward symptoms.

A Precision-Engineered Dietary Overhaul – Based on his genetic profile and metabolic markers, AI designed a heart-healthy diet rich in omega-3s, plant-based polyphenols, and anti-inflammatory foods that lowered arterial plaque buildup and improved circulation.

Stress Management for Cardiovascular Protection – The program pinpointed chronic cortisol spikes as a hidden contributor to heart strain, leading Mark to adopt guided meditation, breathwork, and biofeedback techniques to control stress levels.

Targeted Supplementation for Heart Health – AI prescribed precise micronutrient support, including CoQ10 for energy production, magnesium for blood pressure regulation, and curcumin for reducing arterial inflammation.

A Heart Rebuilt, A Future Reclaimed

Within months, Mark felt like a new man – his blood pressure dropped, arterial inflammation subsided, and his heart was no longer under silent stress. He restored energy levels – no more unexplained fatigue or shortness of breath. He improved heart rate variability and stress resilience – his AI-driven program had retrained his nervous system to promote cardiovascular health. Most powerfully, he had quite literally averted a life-threatening heart attack before it ever had a chance to occur. AI had intervened before disaster struck, allowing him to rewrite his future and extend his health span.

AI is the Future of Preventative Medicine

Mark's journey proves that the greatest breakthroughs in healthcare aren't just about treating disease – they're about preventing it before it ever manifests. Mark didn't just improve his health – he changed the trajectory of his life. AI gave him a second chance before he ever needed one, proving that the future of medicine is not just about living longer, but living smarter.

For Biohacking and AI-Guided Anti-Aging Therapies

In the realm of biohacking and AI-guided anti-aging therapies, the next generation of innovations includes real-time optimization of aging processes. Peptide Therapy – AI helps identify specific peptides that optimize hormone levels, muscle recovery, and cognitive function. Stem Cell Rejuvenation – AI-driven stem cell research is paving the way for regenerative medicine. Cryotherapy and heat therapy – AI now tracks recovery data to customize cold and heat exposure for optimal cellular repair and performance.

Technological Innovations in Age Management

Advancements in technology, such as wearable health devices, telemedicine, and personalized medicine, are transforming how we approach aging. A chapter on this topic can highlight current and emerging technologies that aid in monitoring health, preventing disease, and promoting longevity.

In the twenty-first century, rapid technological advancements are reshaping our approach to aging. Innovations such as wearable health devices, telemedicine, and personalized medicine are not only enhancing our ability to monitor health and prevent disease but also promoting longevity and improving the quality of life for older adults.

Wearable Health Devices: Wearable technology has become increasingly popular, providing older adults with tools to monitor vital signs and activity levels, thereby promoting active and healthy lifestyles.

Fitness Trackers and Smartwatches: Devices such as fitness trackers and smartwatches monitor physical activity, heart rate, sleep patterns, and other health metrics. These devices encourage users to maintain an active lifestyle and provide data that can be shared with healthcare providers for personalized care plans.

Medical Alert Systems: Advanced medical alert systems

now come equipped with features like fall detection, GPS tracking, and emergency communication capabilities, ensuring that older adults can receive immediate assistance when needed.

Telemedicine: Telemedicine has become a vital tool in providing healthcare services to older adults, especially those with mobility challenges or residing in remote areas.

Virtual Consultations: Through virtual consultations, telehealth platforms now allow patients to connect with doctors in real-time via video calls, reducing the need for in-person visits and allowing for timely medical advice. This approach has been particularly beneficial during the COVID-19 pandemic, ensuring continuity of care while minimizing exposure risks.

Remote Monitoring: Remote patient monitoring systems collect health data from patients in real-time, allowing healthcare providers to track conditions such as hypertension, diabetes, and heart disease, and to intervene promptly when necessary.

Personalized Medicine: Advancements in genomics and biotechnology have paved the way for personalized medicine, tailoring healthcare to individual genetic profiles.

Genetic Testing: Genetic tests can identify predispositions to certain diseases, enabling proactive management and personalized treatment plans.

Pharmacogenomics: Understanding how an individual's genetic makeup affects their response to medications allows for the selection of the most effective drugs with minimal side effects, enhancing treatment efficacy.

Smart Home Technologies

Smart home technologies are enhancing the ability of older adults to age in place by creating safer and more supportive living environments.

Home Automation: Smart home devices can automate lighting, temperature control, and security systems, making daily living more convenient and reducing the risk of accidents.

Health Monitoring: Innovations such as the Interactive Care Platform (I-Care) connect older adults experiencing cognitive impairment to their family members who live apart, supporting the completion of important daily activities.

Artificial Intelligence and Robotics

Artificial intelligence (AI) and robotics are playing increasingly significant roles in age management.

Artificial Intelligence and Robotics in Age Management: Case Studies

Artificial intelligence (AI) and robotics are increasingly integral to age management, offering innovative solutions to enhance the quality of life for older adults. The following case studies illustrate the practical applications and benefits of these technologies in elder care.

As dementia rates continue to rise, caregivers and healthcare professionals face increasing challenges in providing consistent, high-quality care to those experiencing cognitive decline. Enter socially assistive robots – a groundbreaking innovation designed to enhance emotional well-being, reduce isolation, and support both dementia patients and their families.

Case Study: "Ka Ka" – The Humanoid Companion for Dementia Care

A recent study explored the deployment of Ka Ka, a humanoid social robot, in the homes of older adults with dementia over a two-week period. The goal? To assess its impact on emotional engagement, social interaction, and caregiver burden.

The results were profound. "Ka Ka" transformed the dementia care experience. Participants who often struggled with isolation and communication found a new companion in Ka Ka. The robot engaged them in gentle conversations, guided memory exercises, and interactive storytelling sessions, leading to noticeable improvements in mood, engagement, and responsiveness. For families caring for a loved one with dementia, the daily emotional and physical toll can be overwhelming. The introduction of Ka Ka provided a much-needed respite, offering companionship and cognitive stimulation that eased caregiver stress. Caregivers reported:

Cognitive Stimulation and Routine Reinforcement

Dementia often disrupts routine and memory recall, making everyday life challenging. Ka Ka assisted in reminding patients to take medication, drink water, and follow daily schedules. Engaging them in memory games and conversational prompts designed to slow cognitive decline. Providing soothing music and relaxation techniques to ease anxiety and restlessness.

The Future of Dementia Care is Smart, Compassionate, and Technologically Driven

Ka Ka's case study proves that socially assistive robots are more than just futuristic gadgets – they are transformative tools in dementia care. Ka Ka marks a pivotal shift in how we address aging, social connection, and emotional care in dementia settings. While technology will never replace human love and touch, it can bridge the gap, offering support, engagement, and dignity to those navigating the challenges of cognitive decline.

AI-Enabled Monitoring Systems in Care Homes: Revolutionizing Resident Safety and Care

As the demand for high-quality elder care rises, innovative technologies like AI-enabled monitoring systems are transforming the way care homes support residents – particularly those with dementia and mobility challenges. One such advancement is the "Ally Cares" system, an AI-powered solution that enhances resident safety, proactive healthcare, and staff efficiency.

Case Study: The "Ally Cares" System – A Game Changer in UK Care Homes

In a UK-based care home, the implementation of Ally Cares marked a significant breakthrough in real-time health monitoring and incident prevention. Unlike traditional reactive approaches, this system used AI-driven analytics to predict risks, detect anomalies, and provide early interventions.

The impact? Safer residents, faster responses, and improved care quality. "Ally Cares" transformed resident safety and well-being. AI-powered fall detection and mobility monitoring. Falls are one of the leading causes of injury in care homes, particularly among elderly residents with limited mobility. Ally Cares utilized motion sensors and behavioral pattern analysis to detect sudden movements or unsteady walking patterns that signaled a risk of falling. Alert staff in real-time if a resident attempted to get out of bed at night or moved in an unsafe manner. Reduce response times dramatically, ensuring immediate assistance when needed.

Early Health Deterioration Detection

By continuously monitoring vital signs, sleep patterns, and subtle behavioral changes, the AI system could identify early warning signs of infections, respiratory distress, or cognitive decline before symptoms became severe. This allowed caregivers to intervene proactively, reducing emergency hospitalizations. Adjust care plans based on real-time health trends.

Improve overall resident well-being with preventive strategies. Enhanced efficiency for care staff. Rather than relying solely on scheduled check-ins, the care team used Ally Cares' real-time alerts and predictive analytics to provide personalized, responsive care.

The Ally Cares system demonstrates that AI isn't here to replace human caregivers – it's here to enhance their ability to provide compassionate, proactive, and efficient care. The future of elder care lies in intelligent, data-driven solutions that allow for safer, more dignified aging. AI monitoring systems like Ally Cares are ushering in a new era where technology and empathy work hand in hand to improve quality of life.

Case Study: ElliQ Companion Robot

The ElliQ companion robot, developed by Intuition Robotics, was introduced into the homes of seniors to promote independence and provide companionship. Unlike traditional voice assistants, ElliQ engages users in proactive conversations, offers health and wellness support, and can send health updates to caregivers. Users reported a decrease in feelings of loneliness and an improvement in mental health, attributing these benefits to the robot's interactive and supportive features. Caregivers also appreciated the timely health alerts, which facilitated better management of their loved ones' well-being.

Case Study: Caspar AI in Senior Housing

Caspar AI implemented an AI-enabled automation system in senior living communities to enhance safety and reduce risks associated with aging. The system automated various aspects of the living environment, such as lighting, climate control, and security, tailored to the residents' routines and preferences. It also monitored daily activities to detect anomalies that might indicate health issues. Residents experienced increased comfort and safety, while staff could focus more on direct care activities, knowing that the AI system provided an additional layer of oversight.

Case Study: Japan's Integration of AI and Robotics

Facing a rapidly aging population and a shrinking labor

force, Japan has turned to AI and robotics to maintain productivity and support its elderly citizens. Robots have been deployed in various sectors, including healthcare, where they assist with tasks ranging from patient care to administrative duties. This integration has helped mitigate the challenges posed by labor shortages, ensuring that the needs of the aging population are met without overburdening the existing workforce.

Together, these case studies underscore how AI and robotics are not just supporting aging populations – they're helping them thrive. By enhancing companionship, monitoring health, improving safety, and addressing labor challenges, these technologies contribute significantly to the well-being and quality of life of older adults. As advancements continue, it is essential to consider ethical implications and ensure equitable access to these innovations, promoting a future where aging populations can thrive with the support of intelligent systems.

AI in Diagnostics

AI algorithms can analyze medical data to assist in early disease detection, risk assessment, and personalized treatment planning. Artificial Intelligence (AI) is revolutionizing medical diagnostics by analyzing complex medical data to assist in early disease detection, risk assessment, and personalized treatment planning. The following case studies illustrate the practical applications and benefits of AI in diagnostics across various medical fields.

AI in Lung Disease Diagnosis

Researchers at Charles Darwin University, in collaboration with United International University and Australian Catholic University, have developed an AI model to diagnose pneumonia, COVID-19, and other lung diseases using lung ultrasound videos. The model analyzes each video frame to identify key lung features and assess patterns, achieving a diagnostic accuracy of 96.57 percent. This AI system utilizes explainable AI techniques, enhancing clinical transparency and aiding in quick and accurate diagnosis. The model's versatility allows for potential training to diagnose additional diseases such as tuberculosis, asthma, and cancer.

AI in Cancer Detection

A UK-based startup, C the Signs, has developed an AI tool that predicts cancer risk by analyzing patients' symptoms and medical records. In a study involving 122,193 patients, the tool demonstrated a 99.3 percent sensitivity in identifying cancer risks. By assisting doctors in identifying high-risk patients, this AI tool facilitates early and more effective treatment, supporting physicians' judgment without replacing it. The company is currently in discussions with the FDA to introduce the tool into the U.S. market.

AI in Prostate Cancer Diagnosis

A study by UCLA researchers evaluated an AI tool called Unfold AI, developed by Avenda Health, for prostate cancer detection. The AI achieved an 84 percent accuracy rate, surpassing the 67 percent accuracy rate of human doctors. Unfold AI uses an algorithm to create 3D cancer estimation maps from clinical data, helping to identify precise cancer margins. This method proved effective in targeting cancer while preserving the prostate gland's functional structures, leading to fewer side effects such as incontinence and impotence.

AI in Medical Imaging

Aidoc, an Israeli technology company, has developed AI algorithms that assist in diagnosing various conditions through medical imaging. Their FDA-approved systems can detect intracranial hemorrhage, pulmonary embolism, and cervical fractures, among other conditions. These algorithms are in use in more than 900 hospitals and imaging centers, including prominent institutions like Yale New

Haven Hospital and Cedars-Sinai Medical Center. By prioritizing potentially critical findings, Aidoc's AI improves patient outcomes by enabling faster diagnosis and treatment.

AI in Histopathological Diagnostics

A study titled "AI-based Anomaly Detection for Clinical-Grade Histopathological Diagnostics" explored the use of AI in detecting anomalies in histopathological images. The AI model was trained on a large dataset of gastrointestinal biopsies and demonstrated high accuracy in identifying a broad spectrum of infrequent pathologies, including rare cancers. This approach facilitates case prioritization, reduces missed diagnoses, and enhances the general safety of AI models in routine diagnostics.

These case studies highlight the transformative potential of AI in medical diagnostics. By leveraging advanced algorithms to analyze complex medical data, AI systems assist healthcare professionals in early disease detection, accurate risk assessment, and personalized treatment planning. As AI technology continues to evolve, its integration into clinical practice holds promise for improving patient outcomes and advancing the field of medicine.

Assistive Robots

Robots are designed to assist with daily activities, provide companionship, and monitor health parameters, enhancing the independence and well-being of older adults.

Assistive robots are increasingly being utilized to support older adults in daily activities, provide companionship, and monitor health parameters, thereby enhancing their independence and well-being. These robots, often referred to as Socially Assistive Robots (SARs), are designed to interact with individuals in a socially meaningful way, offering both functional assistance and emotional support. The following case studies illustrate the practical applications and benefits of assistive robots in elder care.

Case Study: Memory Game with a Socially Assistive Robot

A study explored the use of a socially assistive robot to play a memory game with older adults. The robot was designed with human-like assistive and social characteristics to determine if these features would result in positive attitudes from the elderly participants. The findings indicated that the participants responded favorably to the robot, engaging actively in the game and exhibiting positive emotional responses. This interaction not only provided cognitive stimulation but also offered social engagement, which is crucial for mental well-being in older adults.

Case Study: Integration of Assistive Robotics in Dementia-Friendly Living Spaces

A feasibility study investigated the integration of assistive therapeutic robotics, wearable sensors, and spatial technology within an intelligent environment tailored for dementia care. The system was designed to support residents without necessitating technical expertise, fostering various activities including robot interactions, medication delivery, physical exercises, and cognitive stimulation through puzzles. Physiological data revealed significant participant engagement during robot interactions, indicating the potential effectiveness of robot-assisted activities in enhancing the quality of life for residents.

Case Study: Paro Therapeutic Robot in Nursing Homes

Paro, a robotic seal developed by Japan's National Institute of Advanced Industrial Science and Technology, was designed as a therapeutic tool for use in hospitals and nursing homes. The robot is programmed to cry for attention and respond to its name, facilitating communication among elderly residents. Experiments showed that Paro facilitated elderly residents communicating with each other, which led to psychological improvements.

Case Study: Lovot Companion Robot

Lovot is a Japanese companion robot designed solely to make users happy. It features over fifty sensors that mimic the behavior of a human baby or small pet, including a 360° camera with a microphone, the ability to distinguish humans from objects, and neotenous eyes. An interactive Lovot Café was opened in Japan, allowing individuals to experience interactions with the robot. Such companion robots have the potential to alleviate feelings of loneliness and social isolation among older adults by providing consistent interaction and emotional support.

Case Study: Handle Anywhere Mobile Robot Arm

A study introduced a mobile robot designed to provide an older adult with a handle anywhere in space, termed "handle anywhere." The robot consists of an omnidirectional mobile base attached to a repositionable handle, aimed at supporting autonomy and reducing the risk of falls among elderly individuals. The study analyzed postural changes in various activities of daily living and developed a methodology to optimally place the handle to provide maximum support at points of most effort. This approach enhances patient mobility and reduces the incidence of falls, contributing to safer aging in place.

These case studies demonstrate the diverse applications and benefits of assistive robots in supporting older adults. By providing cognitive stimulation, assisting with daily activities, offering companionship, and enhancing mobility, assistive robots contribute significantly to the independence and well-being of the elderly population. As technology advances, the integration of assistive robots into elder care holds promise for addressing the challenges associated with aging and improving the quality of life for older adults.

Remote Monitoring Enhances Chronic Disease Management

A study involving older adults with chronic heart failure utilized remote monitoring devices to track vital signs such as blood pressure and weight. The data was transmitted to healthcare providers, allowing for timely interventions. The results demonstrated a significant reduction in hospital readmissions and improved patient outcomes.

Telemedicine Improves Access to Care in Rural Areas

In rural communities with limited access to healthcare facilities, telemedicine initiatives provided virtual consultations and remote monitoring services to older adults. This approach led to improved management of chronic conditions, increased patient satisfaction, and reduced travel burdens for patients.

Personalized Medicine in Cancer Treatment

An older patient diagnosed with cancer underwent genetic testing to identify specific mutations driving the disease. Based on the genetic profile, a targeted therapy was selected, resulting in a favorable response and minimal side effects compared to traditional chemotherapy.

Embracing Technology for Healthy Aging

Technological innovations are transforming age management by providing tools that enhance health monitoring, facilitate access to care, and enable personalized interventions. As these technologies continue to evolve, they hold the promise of not only extending lifespan but also improving the quality of life for older adults, allowing them to age with dignity, independence, and vitality.

We are moving toward an era where one-size-fits-all medicine is being replaced by personalized, AI-driven health strategies. With the integration of wearable health tech, genetic testing, and biohacking tools, the potential for radically extending health span and lifespan is closer than ever.

AI and data-driven medicine will continue to evolve, making precision longevity treatments more accessible. By leveraging technology, individuals can take proactive control of their health and slow down aging at a molecular level. The key to longevity isn't just living longer – it's living healthier, with a high quality of life at every stage.

Longevity is no longer a distant dream – it's unfolding in real time, becoming more personal, intelligent, and attainable every day. But here's the most important truth: no technology, no test, no algorithm can replace the power of you – your daily choices, your mindset, your willingness to keep learning and growing. AI can offer insights. Science can extend possibility. But you are still the driver of your journey.

Let this chapter be your reminder: the future isn't something to fear – it's something you get to shape, one choice at a time.

One decision, one habit, one brave step at a time. The tools may be smarter, but the wisdom still lives in you. And that is the true heart of longevity.

CHAPTER 13:
BUILDING YOUR PERSONALIZED LONGEVITY PLAN FOR A HEALTHIER FUTURE

*"Your future health is the result of the choices
you make today – start building your best life now."*
— Maria L. Ellis, BBA, MBA

You've made it. Not just to the end of a book, but to the beginning of a new way of living.

When you first picked this up, you may have been curious – or maybe you were searching. Searching for more energy, more clarity, more connection, more time. You've walked beside Sofia through reinvention, stretched with Emily in pursuit of renewal, reconnected with Lorraine's wisdom, and laughed – and cried – with Elena's transformation. And now, here you are – with the knowledge, the tools, and most importantly, the belief that a vibrant, purpose-filled life is not behind you... it's ahead.

So now the question becomes: What will you do with everything you've discovered?

Build Your Personalized Longevity Plan

This is what it all leads to: the chance to turn stories, insights, and science into a simple plan that fits your life.

Start small. Don't aim for a total life overhaul. Instead, choose one area to focus on this month. Here's a gentle road map to help:

Step 1: Choose Your Pillar

Which area needs your attention most right now? Nutrition, movement, sleep, stress relief,
social connection, cognitive growth, purpose, and joy.

Step 2: Make It Tangible

Write down one small habit you'll begin today. Not perfect – just possible. Add greens to lunch, walk for ten minutes, meditate for three minutes, call one friend this week, start a new book or class, journal before bed.

Step 3: Track How You Feel

Notice the shifts – not just in your body, but in your spirit. Keep a simple journal or voice memo. Are you more clear-headed? More energized? More engaged?

Step 4: Layer Gently

Once that habit becomes second nature, stack another one. Bit by bit, you're building a life that supports your longevity goals. It's not about pressure – it's about momentum.

This is Your Legacy, Too

You may not be a billionaire biohacker or a Silicon Valley scientist, but that's not what longevity requires. You may not want to live to 150. But what you do want – what you deserve – is a life that feels deeply alive, regardless of your age. That's what you're creating here: not just more years, but better years.

You are now the architect of your next chapter. You've learned how to nourish, protect, and renew your body and mind. You've explored emerging therapies and timeless wisdom. You've reimagined what it means to age – and, perhaps, to begin again.

So breathe that in. Own it. Because your longevity plan

isn't just about how long you live – it's about how fully you show up for the moments that matter.

You're not finished. You're just getting started. Now, go live it.

A Tailored Approach to Longevity

No two people age the same way, which is why a personalized longevity plan is essential for maximizing health and lifespan. With the knowledge gained from this book, it's time to put together a comprehensive, customized strategy that fits your unique body, lifestyle, and goals.

This chapter provides a step-by-step guide to designing a personalized longevity blueprint, integrating science-backed habits, cutting-edge technology, and real-life experiences from individuals who have successfully implemented their own longevity strategies.

To begin, take stock of your current health and lifestyle – this is the foundation for optimizing your well-being. This process involves comprehensive medical evaluations, leveraging wearable technology for continuous monitoring, and identifying specific areas that require targeted interventions.

Step 1: Assessing Your Current Health and Lifestyle Consider the following:

Medical Checkups and Biomarker Testing – Start with a full-body assessment, including blood tests, hormone levels, and inflammation markers.

Wearable Technology and Data Tracking – Use devices like the Oura Ring, continuous glucose monitors (CGMs), and fitness trackers to understand your body's unique rhythms.

Identify Your Weakest Link – Where are you struggling most? Is it sleep? Stress? Metabolism? Start there.

Below are case studies illustrating each of these components:

Case Study: Comprehensive Biomarker Assessment for Preventive Health

A forty-five-year-old individual underwent a full-body assessment, including extensive blood tests to evaluate various biomarkers such as lipid profiles, hormone levels, and inflammation markers. The results revealed elevated levels of C-reactive protein (CRP), indicating systemic inflammation, and an imbalance in thyroid hormones suggestive of subclinical hypothyroidism. Based on these findings, the healthcare provider recommended dietary modifications, initiation of anti-inflammatory supplements, and thyroid hormone replacement therapy. Subsequent testing after six months showed normalized CRP levels and improved thyroid function, demonstrating the effectiveness of targeted interventions guided by biomarker testing.

Case Study: Utilizing Continuous Glucose Monitoring for Metabolic Health

A thirty-four-year-old marketing executive experienced persistent fatigue and energy crashes throughout the day. To gain insights into her body's glucose dynamics, she utilized a continuous glucose monitor (CGM). The CGM data revealed significant blood sugar spikes following the consumption of certain carbohydrate-rich meals. Armed with this information, she adjusted her diet to include more balanced macronutrient ratios and opted for low-glycemic index foods. Over the next few months, she reported sustained energy levels, reduced fatigue, and even a fifteen-pound weight loss, highlighting the impact of personalized data tracking on health outcomes.

Case Study: Addressing Sleep Deficiency to Enhance Overall Health

A fifty-year-old male with a demanding job reported chronic sleep deprivation, averaging only five hours of sleep per night. He also experienced elevated stress levels and struggled with weight management. Recognizing sleep as his weakest link, he implemented a structured sleep hygiene program, which included establishing a consistent bedtime routine, minimizing screen exposure before bed, and creating a restful sleep environment. After three months, he increased his average sleep duration to seven hours per night. Consequently, he noticed a significant reduction in stress levels, improved mood, and a gradual weight loss of ten pounds, underscoring the interconnectedness of sleep with other aspects of health.

These case studies demonstrate the importance of comprehensive health assessments, the utilization of wearable technology for personalized data insights, and the strategic targeting of specific health challenges. By adopting a tailored approach to health management, individuals can effectively address their unique needs and enhance their overall well-being.

Step 2: Nutrition and Fasting Strategies for Longevity consider the following:

Intermittent Fasting and Meal Timing – Adopting a fasting protocol to enhance autophagy and cellular repair.

Anti-Inflammatory and Brain-Boosting Diet – Prioritizing omega-3s, polyphenols, and fiber supports metabolic and cognitive health.

Personalized Nutrition Based on DNA Testing – Genetic insights can tailor your diet to prevent disease and optimize metabolism.

The right nutrition and fasting strategies can powerfully influence how you age – from the inside out.

Case Study: Enhancing Autophagy through Intermittent Fasting

A fifty-two-year-old woman adopted a 16:8 intermittent fasting regimen, fasting for sixteen hours and consuming meals within an eight-hour window daily. This approach aimed to stimulate autophagy – a cellular process that removes damaged components and supports cellular repair. After six months, she reported increased energy levels, improved mental clarity, and a ten-pound weight loss. Her physician noted improved biomarkers, including reduced fasting blood glucose and decreased inflammatory markers. These benefits are consistent with research suggesting that intermittent fasting can enhance autophagy and promote health span.

Case Study: Prioritizing Omega-3s, Polyphenols, and Fiber

A sixty-year-old man concerned about cognitive decline and metabolic health transitioned to a diet rich in omega-3 fatty acids, polyphenols, and dietary fiber. He incorporated fatty fish, berries, leafy greens, nuts, and whole grains into his meals. After one year, cognitive assessments showed improved memory and executive function. Additionally, his lipid profile improved, with increased HDL cholesterol and decreased LDL cholesterol levels. These outcomes align with studies indicating that such nutrients support metabolic and cognitive health by reducing inflammation and oxidative stress.

Case Study: Tailoring Diet through Genetic Insights

A forty-five-year-old woman underwent genetic testing to identify predispositions affecting her metabolism and nutrient processing. The results revealed variations in genes related to lipid metabolism and caffeine sensitivity. Based on these insights, a dietitian recommended she reduce saturated fat intake and limit caffeine consumption. Over six months, she experienced improved energy levels, a 5 percent reduction in body weight, and normalized blood pressure. This case illustrates how personalized nutrition, guided by genetic information, can effectively prevent disease and optimize metabolism.

These case studies demonstrate the potential benefits of tailored nutrition and fasting strategies in promoting longevity and overall health.

Step 3: Fitness and Movement Optimization

Consider the following:

Strength Training for Longevity – Incorporate resistance exercises to maintain muscle mass and bone density.

Zone 2 Cardio and High-Intensity Intervals – Balancing low-intensity endurance work with occasional bursts of intensity improves heart health.

Mobility and Recovery Practices – Yoga, foam rolling, and stretching prevent injuries and keep joints healthy.

Sleep, Recovery, and Stress Management

Custom Sleep Routine Based on Circadian Rhythms – Aligning sleep cycles with natural body rhythms enhances deep sleep.

Breathwork, Meditation, and Mindfulness – Techniques like box breathing and guided meditation reduce stress and slow aging.

Technology-Assisted Recovery – Using red light therapy, compression therapy, and infrared saunas enhances rejuvenation.

Optimizing fitness and movement is crucial for promoting longevity and maintaining overall health. The following case studies illustrate the benefits of various exercise strategies, including strength training, Zone 2 cardio combined with high-intensity intervals, and mobility and recovery practices.

Case Study: Resistance Training Enhances Muscle Mass and Reduces Mortality Risk

A sixty-five-year-old woman concerned about age-related muscle loss and bone density decline began a strength training program, engaging in resistance exercises twice weekly. Over a six-month period, she experienced significant improvements in muscle mass and strength. Research indicates that strength training is associated with a 10 to 17 percent lower risk of all-cause mortality, cardiovascular disease, total cancer, diabetes, and lung cancer.

Case Study: Balancing Endurance and Intensity for Heart Health

A fifty-year-old man aiming to improve his cardiovascular health incorporated a combination of Zone 2 cardio and high-intensity interval training (HIIT) into his weekly routine. He performed Zone 2 cardio sessions, such as brisk walking or light jogging, three times a week, maintaining a heart rate that allowed for comfortable conversation. Additionally, he included two weekly HIIT sessions, consisting of short bursts of intense activity followed by recovery periods. After several months, he reported enhanced endurance and overall fitness. Studies suggest that HIIT may be superior for improving mobility, with significant gains in peak oxygen uptake (VO_2peak) achieved after long-interval HIIT.

Step 4: Mobility and Recovery Practices

A fifty-five-year-old man experiencing joint stiffness and occasional muscle soreness integrated yoga and stretching exercises into his fitness regimen. He attended yoga classes twice a week and dedicated time to stretching and foam rolling on alternate days. Over time, he noticed improved flexibility, reduced discomfort, and a decreased incidence of injuries. Recovery practices like stretching and yoga help prevent injuries, protect your joints, and keep you moving with ease.

These case studies underscore the importance of a balanced exercise program that includes strength training, cardiovascular conditioning, and mobility work. Such a comprehensive approach supports longevity by enhancing physical function, reducing disease risk, and promoting overall well-being.

Step 5: Mindset, Social Connection, and Purpose

Building a Longevity-Oriented Community – Surround yourself with people who support your goals.

Finding Purpose in Aging – Engage in meaningful activities that keep you mentally sharp and emotionally ful-filled.

Continuous Learning and Growth – Learning new skills and pursuing passions keeps the brain engaged.

Cultivating a positive mindset, fostering social connections, and pursuing purposeful activities are essential components of longevity and well-being. The following case studies illustrate how individuals and communities have successfully implemented strategies in these areas:

As we conclude this journey into longevity, one truth becomes clear: longevity is not just about extending life – it's about enriching the life we have. By integrating the latest breakthroughs in personalized health, regenerative medicine, and bioenergetics, we can optimize our vitality and well-being.

One emerging innovation, Mitopure® by Timeline Longevity, has been shown to enhance mitochondrial function and boost cellular energy.

In the pursuit of longevity and optimal health, managing exposure to artificial light and harnessing therapeutic light technologies have become focal points. TrueDark's blue light-blocking glasses and TrueLight's red light therapy devices are two innovations designed to address these aspects.

TrueDark Blue Light-Blocking Glasses

Modern lifestyles often involve prolonged exposure to artificial blue light emitted by screens and LED lighting. While blue light during daytime can enhance alertness, excessive exposure, especially during evening hours, can disrupt circadian rhythms and impair sleep quality. TrueDark's blue light-blocking glasses are engineered to filter out specific wavelengths of blue light, thereby mitigating these adverse effects.

By wearing these glasses in the evening, users can reduce the suppression of melatonin production, a hormone crucial for sleep regulation. This practice supports the body's natural sleep-wake cycle, potentially leading to improved sleep quality and overall well-being. Additionally, minimizing blue light exposure may reduce eye strain and fatigue associated with prolonged screen time.

TrueLight Red Light Therapy Devices

Red light therapy, also known as photobiomodulation, involves the application of specific wavelengths of red and near-infrared light to the skin. This therapy has been associated with various health benefits, including enhanced cellular repair, increased collagen production, and reduced inflammation.

TrueLight's red light devices deliver targeted wavelengths that promote skin renewal, reduce inflammation, and support recovery. Regular use of these devices may improve skin texture, reduce the appearance of wrinkles, and accelerate healing processes. Moreover, red light therapy has been explored for its potential to alleviate muscle soreness and support recovery after physical activity.

Integrating Light Management into Daily Life

Incorporating TrueDark blue light-blocking glasses and TrueLight red light therapy into daily routines offers a proactive approach to managing light exposure. By reducing harmful artificial light in the evening and utilizing therapeutic light wavelengths, individuals can support their circadian rhythms, enhance sleep quality, and promote skin health.

As with any health intervention, individual experiences may vary. It's advisable to consult with healthcare professionals to determine the most appropriate strategies for your specific needs.

Embarking on a journey toward a longer, healthier life is a dynamic and personalized endeavor. By integrating evidence-based strategies, individualized data, and a proactive mindset, you can actively influence your aging process and enhance your overall well-being.

Start Small: Focus on One Change at a Time

Initiating your longevity plan with manageable steps is crucial. Concentrate on implementing one change at a time, such as incorporating a daily walk into your routine or adjusting your diet to include more whole foods. This approach fosters sustainable habits and prevents overwhelm, setting a solid foundation for long-term health improvements.

Track Your Progress and Make Adjustments as Needed

Regular monitoring of your progress allows you to assess the effectiveness of your strategies. Utilize tools like journals, apps, or wearable devices to record your activities, dietary intake, and health metrics. This data-driven approach enables you to make informed adjustments, ensuring that your plan remains aligned with your evolving needs and goals.

Stay Curious, Adaptable, and Engaged in Your Health Journey

Maintaining a sense of curiosity and adaptability is essential. Stay informed about emerging health research and be open to experimenting with new strategies that may benefit your well-being. Engage actively in your health journey by seeking knowledge, asking questions, and embracing change. This proactive attitude empowers you to make decisions that support your longevity and quality of life.

As we conclude this journey into longevity, one truth becomes clear: longevity is not just about extending life – it's about enriching the life we have. Every small change, every intentional decision, and every embrace of new technology contributes to a future where we don't just live longer, but we live better.

Throughout this book, we have explored the science of

aging, the breakthroughs in longevity research, and the practical ways to apply these findings to our daily lives. We have seen how nutrition, exercise, mindset, and community all play crucial roles in shaping our health span. We have also delved into cutting-edge innovations – AI-driven health optimization, gene therapies, and biohacking strategies – that are reshaping the future of aging.

But at the heart of all these strategies lies a simple yet profound principle: the power to shape our longevity is in our hands. We are no longer passive participants in the aging process; we are active architects of our future health and vitality.

Your Longevity Action Plan: Moving Forward with Purpose. As you embark on your longevity journey, keep these guiding principles in mind:

Commit to Lifelong Learning – The science of longevity is constantly evolving. Stay informed, explore new advancements, and remain open to adapting your approach as new discoveries emerge.

Listen to Your Body – Personalized longevity is about understanding what works best for you. Monitor your health, track progress, and make adjustments to optimize your well-being.

Cultivate a Longevity-Focused Community – Surround yourself with like-minded individuals who inspire and support your health goals. A strong network makes long-term success more achievable.

Prioritize Purpose and Joy – True longevity goes beyond physical health. Nurture meaningful relationships, engage in fulfilling activities, and cultivate a mindset that brings happiness and purpose to your life.

One Grand Story: Margaret's New Beginning at Eighty-Two

When Margaret first started building her longevity plan, she wasn't trying to reverse time – she was simply trying to stop feeling invisible.

At eighty-two, she had lived through joy and heartbreak, raised three children, lost her husband, and spent decades taking care of everyone but herself. Her days had grown quiet, her joints stiff, her energy low. Her doctor told her she was "doing fine for her age," but Margaret didn't want to settle for fine. She wanted to feel alive again.

So she made a decision: to treat this next season of life as a beginning – not an ending.

She began with food – simple shifts like adding leafy greens, cutting back on sugar, and drinking more water. Within weeks, her bloating eased, her skin looked brighter, and her moods began to stabilize. Then she added movement – gentle yoga at home and short walks outside. Not to burn calories, but to breathe deeper, stretch wider, and feel her body moving again.

Next came sleep – no more falling asleep in front of the TV. She created a soothing bedtime routine and woke up more refreshed than she had in years.

Then, Margaret did something bold. She joined a storytelling group at her local library. Every week, she gathered with others to share pieces of her life – her loves, her regrets, her wisdom. For the first time in a long time, she felt heard. Seen. Needed.

The transformation wasn't instant. It was quiet and steady. But one day, she looked in the mirror and said aloud, "I know this woman. And I like her."

Margaret didn't need to become someone else. She just needed to return to herself. Her personalized longevity plan wasn't about perfection. It was about remembering that she still had a voice, a body, a purpose – and the power to shape her own story.

Margaret's story is your reminder: the steps may be small, but the shift they create can be profound.

And now, it's your turn. Your longevity blueprint is waiting to be lived. One day. One choice. One beautiful beginning at a time.

A Life Well-Lived

Aging is inevitable, but how we age is a choice. By embracing these strategies, you're not just aging – you're redefining it. Whether you are fifty, sixty, or eighty, it is never too late to begin your longevity journey.

As we conclude this exploration into the science and art of longevity, it's essential to recognize that the journey toward a longer, healthier life is both personal and dynamic. By embracing evidence-based strategies, staying informed about emerging research, and maintaining a proactive and adaptable mindset, you can significantly influence your health span – the period of life spent in good health. Remember, small, consistent changes can lead to profound improvements over time. Stay curious, remain engaged in your health journey, and continue to seek out knowledge that empowers you to make informed decisions. Your commitment to understanding and optimizing your well-being is a testament to the remarkable potential of human resilience and the pursuit of a fulfilling life.

Imagine a future where you wake up each day feeling energized, engaged, and inspired. A future where you are not limited by age but empowered by knowledge and action. That future begins today. Thank you for joining me on this journey. May we all live not just longer lives, but lives filled with passion, purpose, and joy. Here's to a future where you don't just survive – but thrive. Because longevity isn't just about more years – it's about better ones.

BONUS CHAPTER: PIONEERS OF LONGEVITY

As humanity stands on the threshold of an unprecedented era of extended life, it is the visionaries – the scientists, entrepreneurs, healers, and innovators – who are lighting the way. Their groundbreaking work is reshaping how we understand aging, health, and the very nature of human potential. In this chapter, we honor these pioneers of longevity, offering brief glimpses into their remarkable contributions. Though their methods range from biotechnology to ancient wisdom, they share one belief: aging is not a destiny, but a frontier to be explored – and extended.

Over the years, I have had the incredible privilege of connecting with some of today's most inspiring leaders and visionaries at the Biohacking Conference – the world's largest and most dynamic event of its kind – led by the unstoppable David Asprey, the "Father of Biohacking." Get ready to meet the trailblazers of longevity, wellness, and consciousness, and discover the bold visions they are bringing into reality.

Dr. Deepak Chopra: The Pioneer of Mind-Body Longevity

"Through consciousness, we unlock not only the secrets to longevity, but the true art of living – and teaching others

to do the same."— Dr. Deepak Chopra

Dr. Deepak Chopra, founder of The Chopra Foundation, has been a transformative leader in the fields of integrative medicine, consciousness, and longevity for over four decades. He bridges ancient wisdom and modern science to offer a holistic model where body, mind, and spirit are deeply interconnected.

Through his many bestselling books, teachings, and global initiatives, Dr. Chopra has inspired millions to understand that lasting health and extended life are not achieved through physical means alone, but through a deeper connection to consciousness, purpose, and inner peace.

Central to Dr. Chopra's philosophy is the idea that our biology is not fixed. Through meditation, mindful living, proper nutrition, emotional balance, and spiritual growth, we can influence genetic expression, reduce inflammation, and slow the aging process at a cellular level. His groundbreaking concept of "radical well-being" emphasizes that true vitality comes from aligning the physical, emotional, mental, and spiritual dimensions of life. In this model, longevity is not simply about adding years to life, but about expanding the richness and fullness of every moment we live.

At the core of Dr. Chopra's vision is a revolutionary truth: aging can be redefined, and human potential is far greater than we once believed. His work invites us to see longevity as a natural outcome of living consciously, nurturing joy, and embracing our intrinsic wholeness. In 2021, I had the privilege of studying directly under Dr. Chopra, completing his program and becoming a Certified Health Instructor. This experience deepened my appreciation for his teachings and reinforced my belief that cultivating inner harmony is one of the most powerful ways to extend both the quality and the length of our lives.

Jirka Rysavy: A Visionary at the Intersection of Consciousness and Longevity

*"When we align mind, body, and spirit, we awaken
the true potential of human evolution." — Jirka Rysavy*

When discussing the future of longevity, one cannot ignore the broader dimensions of human potential – beyond the physical body alone. Jirka Rysavy, CEO and Chairman of Igniton and Executive Chairman of Gaia, embodies this holistic vision. His work emphasizes that longevity is not merely an extension of lifespan, but an expansion of consciousness, health, and human capacity.

His newest venture, Igniton, explores cutting-edge developments at the nexus of consciousness expansion and technological innovation. Though still emerging, Igniton reflects Rysavy's commitment. Jirka Rysavy's life's work offers a critical reminder: longevity is not only about living longer, but about living better, with higher consciousness, deeper meaning, and greater vitality.

In an era where many focus solely on the biology of aging, Rysavy invites us to expand our view – to include the mind, spirit, and heart in our longevity journey. His vision aligns perfectly with the next chapter of human potential, where lifespan and "mindspan" grow together, unlocking a more profound experience of life on Earth.

Dr. Joe Dispenza: Unlocking Human Potential Through Mind and Energy

*"The power to heal and transform lies within the thoughts you
think and the emotions you feel." — Dr. Joe Dispenza*

Dr. Joe Dispenza is a renowned neuroscientist, educator, and bestselling author whose groundbreaking work bridges the worlds of neuroscience, epigenetics, meditation, and quantum physics. His research focuses on the extraordinary power of the mind to influence the body's biology and unlock the potential for self-healing, transformation, and extended vitality.

Through his workshops, retreats, and writings, Dispenza teaches that thoughts, emotions, and beliefs can reshape our genetic expression, alter brain chemistry, and activate regenerative processes. His methods empower individuals to break free from old habits, overcome disease, and create a healthier, more vibrant future through the deliberate practice of meditation, emotional regulation, and mental rehearsal.

At the core of Dr. Dispenza's message is the idea that by changing our internal environment – our thoughts, feelings, and perceptions – we can literally change our external reality.

"Longevity, he teaches, isn't just about genetics or environment – it's shaped by the thoughts and emotions we choose daily."

Dr. Rollin McCraty: The Ultimate Heart Whisperer

"The heart is not just a pump – it is the gateway to resilience, vitality, and a longer, more meaningful life." — Dr. Rollin McCraty

Dr. Rollin McCraty, Director of Research at the HeartMath Institute, has devoted his life's work to understanding the profound role the heart plays in human health, emotional regulation, and longevity. His research reveals the heart is more than a pump – it's an information-processing center influencing the brain, immunity, and even gene expression.

Through his leadership at HeartMath, Dr. McCraty has helped develop practical tools and technologies that teach individuals how to access a state of "heart coherence," a state of inner balance that supports optimal health and resilience.

One of Dr. McCraty's major contributions is the scientific validation of the heart's electromagnetic field and its connection to emotional well-being and physiological performance. His research reveals that when we shift into positive emotional states like gratitude, compassion, and appreciation, our heart rhythms become more harmonious, triggering beneficial effects throughout the body. This "heart-brain connection" is now recognized as a critical key to managing stress, enhancing cognitive function, and ultimately extending both the quality and the quantity of life.

At the heart of Dr. McCraty's vision is a simple yet transformative truth: by learning to listen to and align with the intelligence of the heart, we can unlock deeper levels of healing, vitality, and human potential. His work reminds us that true longevity is not just about extending years – it is about living those years with greater emotional richness, resilience, and connection to ourselves and the world around us.

Peter Crone: The Mind Architect of Freedom and Vitality

"When you free the mind, the body follows –
and true vitality begins." — Peter Crone

Peter Crone, widely known as "The Mind Architect," is a groundbreaking thought leader in the fields of human potential, health, and consciousness. His work focuses on the fundamental truth that much of human suffering – and the limits we experience around health, relationships, and success – are rooted not in external circumstances, but in the subconscious beliefs and mental constructs we unknowingly carry. Crone's mission is to help people transcend these invisible prisons, creating new mental architectures that foster true freedom, peace, and expanded vitality.

Through his coaching, speaking engagements, and public teachings, Peter Crone guides individuals to identify and dissolve the deep-seated patterns of fear, lack, and unworthiness that restrict human flourishing. By releasing these subconscious patterns, people shift from stress to authentic well-being and resilience. His insights demonstrate that the mind-body connection is a powerful key to health and longevity: when the mind is freed from survival-driven thinking, the body naturally follows with healing, restoration, and energetic renewal.

At the heart of Peter Crone's philosophy is the belief that true freedom is not something we achieve by fixing external situations – it is an internal realization available to anyone willing to rethink their relationship with life. In the context of longevity, Crone offers a profound perspective: that releasing psychological and emotional stress is just as critical as nutrition, exercise, or medicine for living a vibrant, expanded life. His work inspires a new paradigm where mental liberation becomes the foundation for human thriving.

Christian Drapeau: Unlocking the Body's Regenerative Power

"The key to longevity lies within – awakening the body's natural ability to heal, renew, and thrive." — Christian Drapeau

Christian Drapeau, a leading scientist and longevity expert, has dedicated his career to exploring the remarkable regenerative capacity of the human body. As the Founder and Chief Science Officer of STEMREGEN, Drapeau has pioneered research into the natural release and function of adult stem cells – a breakthrough that has reshaped the conversation around healing, aging, and longevity. He believes the body already holds the tools for repair and rejuvenation – and that stem cell activation is the key.

Through his research, Drapeau has demonstrated how supporting the body's natural stem cell production can significantly enhance tissue repair, boost immune function, and slow the degenerative processes associated with aging. STEMREGEN, his latest innovation, is a nutraceutical product specifically designed to stimulate the release of the body's own stem cells, offering a natural and accessible approach to cellular renewal. This strategy empowers individuals to take an active role in maintaining their health, promoting resilience from the inside out.

At the heart of Christian Drapeau's work is a profound optimism about the human body's ability to heal itself when given the right support. His contributions are forging a new pathway in the field of longevity – one that honors the body's internal wisdom and leverages nature's own regenerative blueprint. I take STEMREGEN on a daily basis as part of my longevity routine and have experienced firsthand the benefits of supporting natural stem cell health. By making stem cell optimization accessible, Drapeau is helping to redefine what is possible for aging gracefully, vibrantly, and naturally.

Ryan Holiday: The Modern Voice of Stoic Wisdom and Resilient Living

"True strength – and true longevity – comes from mastering what is within your control." — Ryan Holiday

Ryan Holiday, best-selling author and creator of The Daily Stoic, has become one of the leading voices in bringing ancient philosophy into the modern conversation on wellness, resilience, and longevity. Through his books, newsletters, and talks, Holiday shares the timeless principles of Stoicism – discipline, courage, wisdom, and justice – as essential tools for navigating life's challenges with grace and strength. In an age often defined by stress and distraction, his work offers a grounded approach to mental and emotional well-being, which are critical components of living a long and meaningful life.

Holiday's philosophy emphasizes that while we cannot control external events, we can always control our perceptions and responses. This core Stoic teaching directly supports mental health, reduces chronic stress, and fosters emotional resilience – factors that modern science increasingly links to better physical health and extended lifespan. By helping individuals cultivate inner strength, emotional balance, and purpose-driven living, Holiday bridges the wisdom of ancient thinkers like Marcus Aurelius and Seneca with today's quest for health, success, and enduring fulfillment.

At the center of Ryan Holiday's message is the idea that true longevity is not just about adding years, but about building a life of virtue, purpose, and peace. His work reminds us that mastering our inner world is perhaps the greatest secret to thriving in the outer world. Through the lens of Stoicism, Holiday invites us to slow down, focus on what truly matters, and live with integrity – a philosophy that promises not only a longer life but a better one.

Naveen Jain: Transforming Health from the Inside Out

"The future of health – and longevity – is personal, precise, and within your control." — Naveen Jain

Naveen Jain, visionary entrepreneur and founder of Viome, is revolutionizing the way we approach health, disease prevention, and longevity. With a passion for solving some of humanity's biggest challenges, Jain's work focuses on decoding the microbiome – the trillions of microorganisms living inside us – to create personalized solutions for optimal health. Through Viome's cutting-edge technology, Jain empowers individuals to understand their unique biological makeup and make precise dietary and lifestyle choices that enhance vitality and extend health span.

Jain's core belief is that chronic diseases, aging, and even many mental health issues are not inevitable – they are preventable and often reversible when we take a proactive and personalized approach. By analyzing gut health, gene expression, and inflammatory markers, Viome offers customized recommendations that help individuals reduce inflammation, optimize metabolism, and strengthen immunity. This level of precision health not only supports disease prevention but lays the foundation for longer, healthier lives rooted in personal empowerment and informed decision-making.

At the heart of Naveen Jain's vision is the idea that health care should be about wellness, not sickness. He challenges outdated models and inspires a new era where technology, biology, and human potential converge to create a future where aging becomes optional. Jain's work reminds us that the future of longevity will not be found in generic solutions, but in personalized, actionable insights that unlock each person's unique pathway to thriving.

Dr. Patrick Porter: Tuning the Brain for Optimal Health and Longevity

"A healthy brain is the gateway to a vibrant life — and with the right tools, we all have the power to access it." — *Dr. Patrick Porter*

Dr. Patrick Porter, founder of BrainTap, Inc., is a leading expert in brainwave entrainment technology and its powerful impact on mental, emotional, and physical health. Through his groundbreaking work, Dr. Porter has shown that by using specific frequencies of light and sound, we can guide the brain into deeply restorative states, promoting healing, reducing stress, enhancing cognitive function, and supporting overall vitality. His innovations in neuroplasticity and brain fitness are helping redefine how we view brain health as a cornerstone of longevity.

BrainTap technology combines guided visualization, light therapy, and sound frequency entrainment to optimize brainwave patterns, allowing users to effortlessly access states of relaxation, focus, and rejuvenation. By regularly engaging the brain in these balanced states, individuals can reduce the harmful effects of chronic stress — one of the greatest accelerators of aging — and enhance their body's natural capacity for repair and resilience. Dr. Porter's work underscores the vital link between mental well-being and physical longevity, offering practical tools to help people thrive in today's fast-paced world.

At the core of Dr. Porter's mission is the belief that true health and extended vitality begin with the brain. His contributions invite us to see the mind not just as a tool for thinking, but as a dynamic, trainable system that, when properly nurtured, can unlock profound healing, enhanced performance, and a longer, more vibrant life. I use Dr. Porter's BrainTap technology and can attest to its powerful benefits – helping me experience deeper relaxation, sharper focus, and a renewed sense of energy. Through BrainTap and his teachings, Dr. Porter is empowering individuals to take control of their mental fitness and, in doing so, create a powerful foundation for lasting health and longevity.

Dr. Daniel Pompa: Leading the Revolution in Cellular Healing

"If you don't heal the cell, you won't heal the body – and true longevity begins at the cellular level." — *Dr. Daniel Pompa*

Dr. Daniel Pompa is a trailblazer in the field of cellular health and wellness, dedicating his career to addressing the root causes of chronic illness, inflammation, and aging. As the founder of The Pompa Program and Health Centers, he has developed groundbreaking strategies focused on true cellular detoxification, mitochondrial health, and the restoration of optimal body function. Dr. Pompa's philosophy is clear: if you don't heal the cell, you can't truly heal the body. His work has empowered thousands to reclaim their health by going beyond surface-level solutions and targeting healing at the deepest cellular level.

Central to Dr. Pompa's approach is the concept of removing cellular toxins, rebalancing hormones, and optimizing the body's innate capacity for self-repair. He emphasizes fasting protocols, advanced nutrition, and lifestyle interventions designed to reduce inflammation, reset cellular energy pathways, and restore resilience. By focusing on the health of the cell, he offers a powerful model for not just overcoming disease but for dramatically improving energy, mental clarity, and longevity. His protocols are particularly vital in today's world, where environmental toxins and chronic stress continually threaten long-term wellness.

At the heart of Dr. Pompa's mission is a belief that vibrant health and extended life are available to anyone willing to address health from the inside out. His work teaches that true longevity is not about suppressing symptoms or chasing trends – it is about restoring the body's natural blueprint for vitality. Through The Pompa Program, he is creating a global movement, inspiring people to take control of their health at the most foundational level and offering real hope for a longer, healthier, more energized life.

Dr. Jason Sonners: Elevating Health Through the Power of Oxygen

"Oxygen isn't just life support – it's the ultimate catalyst for healing, renewal, and longevity." — *Dr. Jason Sonners*

Dr. Jason Sonners, a pioneering expert in Hyperbaric Oxygen Therapy (HBOT) and a key leader at OxyHealth, is revolutionizing the role of oxygen in health, healing, and longevity. With a background in chiropractic care, functional medicine, and rehabilitation, Dr. Sonners integrates HBOT as a cornerstone therapy for enhancing the body's natural regenerative abilities. His work highlights how oxygen, when used therapeutically under pressure, can dramatically accelerate recovery, reduce inflammation, and stimulate cellular repair – offering a safe and powerful method to support long-term vitality.

Through his clinics and research, Dr. Sonners shows that HBOT isn't just for injuries – it's a tool for longevity. It can optimize brain health, improve immune function, increase energy production at the mitochondrial level, and even activate dormant stem cells. His protocols help people manage chronic illnesses, prevent age-related decline, and enhance overall performance. In a world where environmental stressors constantly challenge our health, HBOT emerges through Dr. Sonners' work as a vital tool for sustaining wellness and promoting a longer, healthier life.

At the heart of Dr. Sonners' philosophy is the understanding that oxygen is not just necessary for survival – it is a transformative resource for thriving. His work invites us to view longevity not only as an extension of years but as a dynamic process of cellular renewal, resilience, and enhanced living. By making cutting-edge HBOT technology accessible and practical, Dr. Jason Sonners is giving individuals a powerful means to unlock their full health potential and age with strength, clarity, and vitality.

Dr. Alberto Villoldo: Bridging Ancient Wisdom and Modern Healing

"Our greatest medicine is the dream we dare to live into reality."
— Dr. Alberto Villoldo

Dr. Alberto Villoldo, a renowned medical anthropologist, psychologist, and shaman, has spent decades studying the healing practices of indigenous cultures in the Amazon and the Andes. His groundbreaking work blends the ancient spiritual traditions of energy medicine with the insights of modern neuroscience and biology, offering a profound vision for human health and longevity. Dr. Villoldo teaches that true healing – and extended vitality – requires not just treating the physical body but also clearing the luminous energy field that surrounds and informs it.

Through his books, teachings, and The Four Winds Society, Dr. Villoldo has introduced countless people to the concept of soul-centered health. He emphasizes the importance of clearing emotional wounds, healing ancestral patterns, and aligning with higher spiritual forces to promote lasting wellness. By integrating techniques such as energy clearing, soul retrieval, and shamanic journeys, he offers a holistic roadmap for aging gracefully, maintaining youthful vitality, and awakening higher states of consciousness that support profound healing.

At the heart of Dr. Villoldo's message is the belief that we are more than our genes and our histories – we are luminous beings capable of rewriting our destinies. His work invites us to step into the role of conscious creators of our own lives, shaping not only our health but our very experience of reality. Through his visionary synthesis of ancient and modern healing traditions, Dr. Villoldo inspires a new paradigm of longevity that honors the body, mind, and spirit as sacred, interconnected forces.

Dr. Jerry Tennant: Harnessing the Power of Voltage for Cellular Healing

"True healing begins not with treating symptoms, but with restoring the energy that powers every cell in the body."
— Dr. Jerry Tennant

Dr. Jerry Tennant, a pioneering physician, researcher, and founder of Tennant Products, has reshaped the field of integrative medicine by uncovering the critical role of voltage in human health and healing. His groundbreaking work in bioenergetic medicine shows that chronic disease and aging are fundamentally problems of low cellular voltage. Dr. Tennant's research reveals that cells need a specific level of electrical energy to function properly, repair themselves, and regenerate – and that restoring voltage at the cellular level can dramatically accelerate healing and extend vitality.

Through his acclaimed Healing is Voltage™ framework, Dr. Tennant developed protocols and technologies that address the root causes of illness by recharging the body's electrical systems. He demonstrates that by optimizing cellular energy through nutrition, hydration, oxygenation, and targeted therapies, we can restore the body's natural ability to heal itself. His approach shifts the focus from symptom management to true cellular repair, offering hope and practical solutions for those facing chronic illness, degeneration, and the effects of aging.

At the heart of Dr. Tennant's work is a revolutionary idea: the body is an electrical system, and healing is an energy process. His teachings inspire a profound shift in how we view health – not merely as the absence of disease but as the presence of vibrant cellular function and energetic balance. By empowering individuals to understand and optimize their body's electrical charge, Dr. Tennant provides a bold, science-based pathway to lasting wellness, resilience, and longevity.

Kasia Urbaniak: Redefining Power and Influence for Women

"Reclaiming your voice isn't just about being heard – it's about unlocking the vitality that comes from living authentically and powerfully." — *Kasia Urbaniak*

Kasia Urbaniak is the founder and CEO of The Academy, a school dedicated to teaching women the foundations of power and influence. Drawing from nearly two decades of experience as a professional dominatrix and seventeen years of training in Taoist alchemy under female mystics in China, Urbaniak offers a unique perspective on power dynamics. Since establishing The Academy in 2013, she has guided thousands of women – including executives, entrepreneurs, artists, and thought leaders – to command authority, influence, and presence in their personal and professional lives.

Through The Academy, Urbaniak challenges the cultural conditioning that often silences women, providing practical tools to break free from the "good girl" paradigm. Her teachings emphasize verbal self-defense, boundary setting, and the art of making bold requests – all aimed at helping women step into leadership roles within their relationships, families, workplaces, and communities.

Incorporating Urbaniak's insights into this longevity book underscores the importance of emotional and psychological health in achieving a long, fulfilling life. She reminds us that vitality isn't just physical – it's the freedom to live authentically, speak boldly, and lead with inner strength.

Dr. Daniel G. Amen: Revolutionizing Brain Health for Lifelong Vitality

"The health of your brain is much more about your actions than your age." — *Dr. Daniel Amen*

Dr. Daniel Amen is a renowned psychiatrist, brain health expert, and founder of Amen Clinics, which houses one of the world's largest databases of functional brain scans. With over 200,000 SPECT scans conducted across 155 countries, Dr. Amen has been instrumental in linking brain health to overall well-being and longevity. His approach emphasizes that by optimizing brain function, individuals can enhance their physical health, emotional balance, and lifespan.

In his book Use Your Brain to Change Your Age, Dr. Amen outlines ten strategies to boost brain health, aiming to help individuals live longer, look younger, and reduce the risk of Alzheimer's disease. These strategies include improving memory, mood, attention, and energy levels, as well as promoting the healing of brain damage due to various factors. By adopting these brain-healthy practices, one can potentially outsmart genetic predispositions and slow down the aging process.

Dr. Amen also highlights the importance of lifestyle choices in maintaining brain health. He advocates for regular exercise, balanced nutrition, adequate sleep, and mental exercises to keep the brain sharp. Moreover, he emphasizes the significance of managing stress and avoiding harmful substances to prevent cognitive decline. His holistic approach underscores that taking care of the brain is paramount to achieving a longer, healthier life. Personally, I have found great value in his teachings and have incorporated several of his products into my daily routine to optimize my brain health and overall well-being. His emphasis on personalized, science-backed strategies has profoundly influenced my approach to wellness, reinforcing the idea that true vitality stems from informed, proactive choices at the cellular level.

Dr. Joseph Mercola: Energizing Health from the Cellular Level Up

"Optimizing your cellular energy is the key to unlocking vibrant

health, longevity, and resilience." — *Dr. Joseph Mercola*

Dr. Joseph Mercola is a pioneering figure in natural health and preventive medicine. As a board-certified osteopathic physician and Fellow of the American College of Nutrition, he has dedicated over four decades to exploring holistic approaches to wellness. Dr. Mercola is the founder of Mercola.com, a widely visited natural health website, and a multiple New York Times bestselling author. His work emphasizes the importance of lifestyle factors – such as nutrition, exercise, and environmental exposures – in influencing health and longevity.

In his recent publication, Your Guide to Cellular Health: Unlocking the Science of Longevity and Joy, Dr. Mercola delves into the role of cellular energy in achieving optimal health. He discusses how modern lifestyle choices and environmental factors can impair mitochondrial function, leading to chronic diseases and premature aging. The book offers actionable insights into diet, detoxification, and lifestyle adjustments aimed at enhancing overall well-being and promoting a longer, healthier life.

Personally, I have found great value in Dr. Mercola's teachings and have incorporated several of his products into my daily routine to optimize my health and longevity. His emphasis on personalized, science-backed strategies has profoundly influenced my approach to wellness, reinforcing the idea that true vitality stems from informed, proactive choices at the cellular level.

"The Exponential Future of Longevity: Breaking the Boundaries of Human Potential"

"You are alive during the most extraordinary time in history – a time when science and technology will give you the tools to live longer, healthier, and more fulfilled than ever before." — *Dr. Peter H. Diamandis, founder of XPRIZE and Fountain Life*

The future of longevity is not unfolding slowly – it is accelerating exponentially. Dr. Peter Diamandis, a visionary entrepreneur and founder of organizations like

XPRIZE and Fountain Life, reminds us that the pace of innovation is doubling every few years. Technologies once thought to be decades away – such as gene therapy, cellular rejuvenation, and predictive AI health platforms – are now arriving faster than ever before. Diamandis believes that the convergence of biotechnology, artificial intelligence, nanotechnology, and regenerative medicine will not just extend life but fundamentally transform it, offering each of us the opportunity to live longer, healthier, and more vibrant lives than any generation before.

One of Diamandis's central ideas is that longevity will be democratized. As technology scales and costs decrease, life-extending interventions will become widely available, not limited to the wealthy elite. His companies are already pioneering affordable precision medicine and longevity clinics that offer comprehensive diagnostics, early disease detection, and regenerative therapies. Accessible, personalized care is crucial – it ensures the longevity revolution benefits everyone, not just a privileged few. Diamandis often emphasizes that taking proactive control of one's health today – through data-driven health tracking, lifestyle optimization, and early adoption of new therapies – is critical to catching the "next bridge" to even more powerful life extension technologies in the coming decades.

Dr. Peter Diamandis advocates for a proactive longevity strategy focused on regular comprehensive health scans, early adoption of cutting-edge therapies, personalized preventive medicine, continuous optimization of diet and exercise, and leveraging exponential technologies to stay ahead of the aging curve. His optimism reframes aging – not as decline, but as a solvable engineering problem. With the exponential growth of scientific discovery, the barriers to living longer are falling away. For those willing to seize the moment, the possibility of seeing 100, 120, or even 180 years of vibrant, purpose-driven life is no longer a fantasy – it is fast becoming a credible, achievable future.

"The New Frontier of Longevity: Reversing Aging and Embracing a Vibrant Future"

"Aging is a disease, and that disease is treatable."
— Dr. David A. Sinclair, Professor of Genetics, Harvard
Medical School, author of Lifespan: Why We Age — and Why We
Don't Have To

In the future of longevity science, the possibilities stretch far beyond merely adding years to our lives — they promise to add vitality, purpose, and mental sharpness as well. Breakthroughs in gene therapy, cellular reprogramming, and AI-driven diagnostics are not just theories; they are emerging realities. Rewinding cells to a younger state — without losing their original function.

These advances suggest that aging itself could become a manageable condition rather than an inevitable decline, offering new hope for living not only longer but stronger.

One of the leading voices in this movement, Dr. David Sinclair, eloquently captures the spirit of this transformation: "Aging is a disease, and that disease is treatable." His work at Harvard Medical School has pushed the boundaries of what we understand about epigenetic reprogramming and cellular resilience. Sinclair's research demonstrates that by targeting the underlying processes of aging — such as DNA damage, mitochondrial decay, and inflammation — we can potentially reverse aspects of aging itself. His optimism is not rooted in fantasy but in rigorous, peer-reviewed science that is rapidly evolving into clinical applications.

As we stand at the cusp of a new era, the call to action is clear: we must not passively accept the traditional trajectory of aging. Instead, we are invited to engage with the extraordinary tools now within our reach. Biohacking, precision supplements, lifestyle optimization, and early adoption of longevity technologies are not luxuries reserved for the elite; they are essential strategies for anyone serious about maximizing their potential lifespan and health span.

Personally, I have embraced this journey by incorporating daily exercise and taking resveratrol, a supplement highly recommended by Dr. Sinclair, as part of my commitment to living a longer, healthier life. The road ahead is filled with promise – but it also demands an open mind, a commitment to learning, and a willingness to evolve alongside the science itself.

New Longevity Technologies

"The future of longevity belongs to those who dare to believe that aging is not a destiny, but a choice – a choice we make every day through knowledge, action, and hope." — Maria L. Ellis, MBA

New longevity technologies being developed today by pioneers like Dr. Peter Diamandis, Dr. David Sinclair, and their colleagues are reshaping what we once thought was the natural human lifespan. From advancements in genetic engineering and cellular reprogramming to AI-driven early diagnostics and regenerative medicine, the dream of dramatically extending human life is no longer confined to science fiction. Companies backed by Diamandis, such as Celularity and Fountain Life, are working to regenerate tissues and organs using placental stem cells, while Sinclair's lab is focused on epigenetic reprogramming – essentially resetting the biological age of cells to a younger, healthier state.

One of the most promising areas of research is the ability to manipulate the "epigenetic clock" – the molecular markers that determine biological age versus chronological age. Dr. Sinclair's experiments in mice have shown that partial cellular reprogramming can reverse aging in certain tissues, restoring sight in blind mice and rejuvenating aged organs. Meanwhile, Diamandis predicts that breakthroughs in gene editing technologies like CRISPR, coupled with AI's ability to personalize medicine at an unprecedented scale, could allow humans to extend their healthy lifespan well beyond today's limits. Their collective vision suggests that we may soon see therapies that repair cellular damage, eliminate senescent cells, and drastically reduce the incidence of age-related diseases.

Will we live to 180 years old? According to Dr. Diamandis, this is not just a possibility – it is a goal being actively pursued. He has famously stated that "the first person who will live to 150 years old has already been born," and possibly, someone alive today could see their life extended even further with the rapid acceleration of these technologies. Skeptics urge caution, noting the complexity of systemic aging. The question is no longer if we can extend human life, but how soon we can democratize access to these revolutionary technologies for all.

The following is a summary of the top five technologies currently leading the charge for extreme longevity.

One of the most exciting frontiers in longevity science is epigenetic reprogramming. Researchers like Dr. David Sinclair have demonstrated that cells can be "reset" to a younger state by altering their epigenetic markers – the chemical tags that regulate gene expression without changing the underlying DNA. This process can reverse age-related decline at the cellular level, opening the door to therapies that may rejuvenate tissues and organs, potentially extending not just lifespan but health span. Early successes in animal studies suggest that restoring youthful gene expression patterns could one day treat degenerative diseases and dramatically slow aging.

Another revolutionary technology is senolytics – drugs and therapies designed to eliminate senescent cells. These so-called "zombie cells" accumulate with age, secreting inflammatory factors that contribute to tissue deterioration, cancer, and chronic diseases. Clearing them from the body has been shown in studies to improve physical function and extend lifespan in mice. Companies like Unity Biotechnology are already testing senolytic drugs in human clinical trials, offering real hope for therapies that target aging at its root.

Stem cell therapies are also transforming the future of

longevity. By harnessing the regenerative power of stem cells, scientists can repair or replace damaged tissues, organs, and even aspects of the immune system. Advances in stem cell banking and regenerative medicine, championed by organizations like Celularity (co-founded by Dr. Peter Diamandis), suggest that in the near future, we may be able to routinely rejuvenate aging bodies by reintroducing young, potent cells to restore function and vitality.

The rise of AI-driven precision medicine is another game-changer. Artificial intelligence can now analyze massive datasets – from genome sequences to biomarker profiles – to create highly personalized health plans. Companies like Fountain Life and Human Longevity Inc. are using AI to detect diseases decades before symptoms appear, offering opportunities for early intervention and prevention that were unimaginable a decade ago. This approach shifts healthcare from reactive to proactive, allowing individuals to optimize their health long before serious problems develop.

Finally, genome editing technologies like CRISPR are giving scientists unprecedented control over the building blocks of life. By precisely editing genes, researchers can correct mutations, turn off harmful genes, or even enhance protective ones. Experimental therapies are already being developed to tackle genetic disorders, but the future could include editing out risk factors for age-related diseases like Alzheimer's, heart disease, and cancer. Combined with other longevity technologies, genome editing holds the potential to drastically extend the quality and duration of human life.

Together, these five breakthroughs form the foundation of the new longevity era. Each is advancing rapidly, and when combined, they promise to redefine what it means to age – and what it means to be human.

Conclusion

As we stand at the edge of a scientific revolution, the

pursuit of longevity is no longer about merely adding years to life – it's about adding life to those years. The technologies now emerging, from epigenetic reprogramming and senolytics to AI-driven diagnostics and genome editing, are transforming how we think about aging and health. Visionaries like Dr. David Sinclair and Dr. Peter Diamandis are not only challenging old assumptions but actively building a future where living well past 100 – even to 150 or 180 years – could be a reality for many.

However, the greatest breakthroughs will not come from technology alone. They will come from our willingness to adapt, to learn, and to proactively engage with these innovations as they unfold. Embracing healthier lifestyles, staying informed about scientific advances, and adopting new interventions when appropriate will be essential to maximizing both our lifespan and our health span.

The road ahead is filled with promise and extraordinary potential. This is more than scientific progress – it's a human awakening. And each of us has the power to choose to be a pioneer in our own longevity story.

ACKNOWLEDGMENTS

Thank you to everyone who helped bring to life, Designing Your Longevity: A Personalized Blueprint for Thriving Longer with Energy, Purpose, and Vitality.

To my family—your unwavering love, support, and belief in me made this journey possible. You have been my foundation and my inspiration through every chapter of my life.

To my friends and mentors, you reminded me that it's never too late to grow, to dream bigger, and to keep learning. Your encouragement fueled my commitment to share this message with the world.

To brilliant scientists, healthcare innovators, and pioneers of longevity, your work continues to inspire hope and transformation for generations to come. Thank you for daring to imagine a better future and for making it real.

And finally, to you—the reader. Thank you for trusting me to walk alongside you as you design your own extraordinary life. May this book be a guiding light as you build a future filled with energy, purpose, and vitality.

With heartfelt gratitude,
Maria L. Ellis, BBA, MBA

ABOUT THE AUTHOR

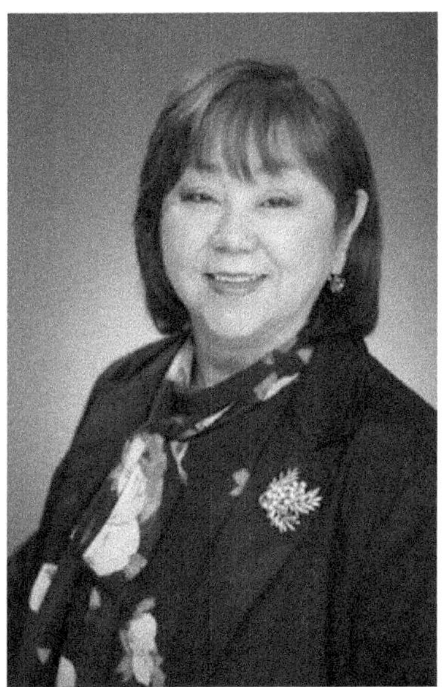

Maria L. Ellis, MBA, is a graduate of the Harvard Business School Owner-President Management Program and
earned her bachelor's degree in business administration as
well as her MBA from the University of Massachusetts in
Amherst. As a former international banker, investment
advisor, and financial planner, Maria has specialized in
converting clients' financial objectives into successful action plans. Maria has both the know-how and the market

contacts, having worked at Bank of America, Citibank, the MONY Group, Northwestern Mutual, Citi Habitats and Keller Williams.

Maria is a Chopra Certified Health Instructor, and she is the bestselling author of the Journey to Wellness, Freedom, and Legacy series, which includes *Achieve Financial Freedom: The Road Map to Financial Success*; *Family Business Legacy Plan: The Ultimate Guide to Creating a Legacy for Your Family without Paying too Much in Taxes*; *Redefining Entrepreneurial Success: A Guide to a Healthy and Holistic Lifestyle*; *Longevity: Reinvent Yourself at Any Age*; *Life on Earth: Poetic Perspectives*; *Golf: A Course in Business: A Few Lessons Golf Can Teach Us about Management and Entrepreneurship;* and *From Operator to Entrepreneur: Unlocking the Power of Visionary Leadership,* and *Stolen Memories: A Journey Through Alzheimer's.*

Maria's background includes board leadership positions at the College of Mount Saint Vincent, the American Association of University Women, and the Virginia Gildersleeve International Fund. Maria is also a pro-bono consultant at the Harvard Business School Club of New York City Community Partners and applies her business skills to a variety of topics, including strategic planning, marketing, finance, governance, and organizational development. Maria is an active member of the Harvard Club and the Genuis Network